PAIN MANAGEMENT - RESEARCH AND TECHNOLOGY

ANTINOCICEPTIVE TOLERANCE TO NSAIDs IN BRAIN LIMBIC AREAS

ROLE OF ENDOGENOUS OPIOID AND CANNABINOID SYSTEMS

PAIN MANAGEMENT - RESEARCH AND TECHNOLOGY

Additional books and e-books in this series can be found on Nova's website under the Series tab.

Pain Management - Research and Technology

Antinociceptive Tolerance to NSAIDs in Brain Limbic Areas

Role of Endogenous Opioid and Cannabinoid Systems

Natia Tsagareli, PhD
Nana Tsiklauri, PhD
and
Merab G. Tsagareli, DSc, PhD

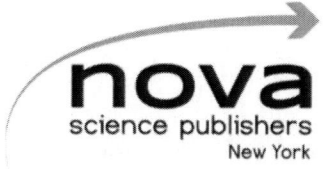
nova science publishers
New York

Copyright © 2021 by Nova Science Publishers, Inc.

All rights reserved. No part of this book may be reproduced, stored in a retrieval system or transmitted in any form or by any means: electronic, electrostatic, magnetic, tape, mechanical photocopying, recording or otherwise without the written permission of the Publisher.

We have partnered with Copyright Clearance Center to make it easy for you to obtain permissions to reuse content from this publication. Simply navigate to this publication's page on Nova's website and locate the "Get Permission" button below the title description. This button is linked directly to the title's permission page on copyright.com. Alternatively, you can visit copyright.com and search by title, ISBN, or ISSN.

For further questions about using the service on copyright.com, please contact:
Copyright Clearance Center
Phone: +1-(978) 750-8400   Fax: +1-(978) 750-4470   E-mail: info@copyright.com.

NOTICE TO THE READER

The Publisher has taken reasonable care in the preparation of this book, but makes no expressed or implied warranty of any kind and assumes no responsibility for any errors or omissions. No liability is assumed for incidental or consequential damages in connection with or arising out of information contained in this book. The Publisher shall not be liable for any special, consequential, or exemplary damages resulting, in whole or in part, from the readers' use of, or reliance upon, this material. Any parts of this book based on government reports are so indicated and copyright is claimed for those parts to the extent applicable to compilations of such works.

Independent verification should be sought for any data, advice or recommendations contained in this book. In addition, no responsibility is assumed by the Publisher for any injury and/or damage to persons or property arising from any methods, products, instructions, ideas or otherwise contained in this publication.

This publication is designed to provide accurate and authoritative information with regard to the subject matter covered herein. It is sold with the clear understanding that the Publisher is not engaged in rendering legal or any other professional services. If legal or any other expert assistance is required, the services of a competent person should be sought. FROM A DECLARATION OF PARTICIPANTS JOINTLY ADOPTED BY A COMMITTEE OF THE AMERICAN BAR ASSOCIATION AND A COMMITTEE OF PUBLISHERS.

Additional color graphics may be available in the e-book version of this book.

Library of Congress Cataloging-in-Publication Data

ISBN: 978-1-53619-814-0

Published by Nova Science Publishers, Inc. † New York

Contents

Preface		vii
List of Abbreviations		ix
Chapter 1	Introduction	1
Chapter 2	Brain Limbic Areas and Pain	5
Chapter 3	Opioid and Cannabinoid Systems	23
Chapter 4	Non-Opioid Tolerance	39
Chapter 5	Antinociceptive Tolerance to NSAIDs in Anterior Cingulate Cortex	45
Chapter 6	Antinociceptive Tolerance to NSAIDs in Insular Cortex	65
Chapter 7	NSAIDs–Induced Antinociception in Central Nucleus of Amygdala	85
Chapter 8	General Discussion	95
Chapter 9	Summary and Conclusion	111
Chapter 10	Methodology (Materials and Methods)	115
References		121

Authors' Contact Information 143

Index 145

PREFACE

The development of pain as a common experience and its treatment is very important, not only where it is caused by injury or inflammation, but also in chronic states where the nerves themselves are damaged. Even though we already know from physiological studies that special pain receptors or nociceptors are responsible for conducting pain sensations to the brain, the phenomenon of pain still remains a medical and social problem. In all cases the development of pain being both disabling and depressing, a multidisciplinary approach is often needed. Pain relief or analgesia can be achieved using a number of different approaches and strategies.

Non-steroidal anti-inflammatory drugs are the most widely used analgesics. They have analgesic, antipyretic, and, at higher doses, anti-inflammatory actions. However, a few recent studies have demonstrated that these non-opioid drugs in the case of their prolonged use, elicit the opioid-like effect, tolerance, which alongside the drug withdrawal syndrome may entail serious adverse effects. The brain limbic system is involved in affective-emotional aspects of pain and here are collected data of the study of brain mechanisms of non-opioid induced antinociceptive tolerance to non-steroidal anti-inflammatory drugs in the "formalin test."

This book provides up-to-date review information and experimental findings of my laboratory young scientists Natia Tsagareli and Nana Tsiklauri by the financial support of the Georgian National Science Foundation. We are grateful to my lab scholars Guliko Gurtskaia and Lia

Nozadze for their professional assistance and owe a special debt to Professor Donald A. Simone from the University of Minnesota, Minneapolis for his valuable notes and comments.

After the Introduction, the next three chapters are devoted to literature reviews on brain limbic areas, opioid and cannabinoid systems, and non-opioid antinociceptive tolerance; the next chapters, – five, six and seven, – describe research data on antinociceptive tolerance to NSAIDs and opioid and cannabinoid mechanisms of attenuation of nociceptive hyperalgesia in the cingulate cortex, insular cortex, and central amygdala, respectively; the chapter number eight deals with discussion, and number nine with summary and conclusions; the last special chapter of Methodology describes experimental materials and methods in detail.

I hope that this book will guide a large reader community through the fascinating world of pain and analgesia research from basic science to pathophysiology and disease. May this source also help to establish interactions between the fundamental and clinical research and the experimentation in drug discovery and development. I wish to thank my both co-authors for their excellent contribution and we will gratefully accept any comments and notes from our readers.

Merab Tsagareli

LIST OF ABBREVIATIONS

ACC	anterior cingulate cortex, rostral ACC (rACC);
AEA	N-arachidonoylethanolamine (anandamide);
AI	anterior insula:
AIC	agranular (anterior) insular cortex;
AMP	adenosine monophosphate;
ANOVA	analysis of variance;
BLA	basolateral amygdala;
BOLD	blood oxygenation level-dependent;
CaMKII	$Ca^{2}+$/calmodulin-dependent protein kinase II
CGRP	calcitonin gene-related peptide;
CB	cannabinoid (receptors), CB1/CB2;
CBD	cannabidiol;
CBP	chronic back pain;
CCI	chronic constriction injury;
CNS	central nervous system;
CeA	central nucleus of amygdala;
COX	cyclo-oxygenase, COX1/COX2;
Coxibs	COX-2 inhibitors;
CRF	corticotrophin-releasing factor;
CRPS	complex regional pain syndrome;
CTOP	D-Phe-Cys-Tyr-D-Trp-Orn-Thr-Pen-Thr-$_{NH2}$
cAMP	cyclic adenosine monophosphate;
DG	dentate gyrus (hippocampus);
DOR	delta opioid receptor;

List of Abbreviations

DH	dorsal hippocampus;
EC	endocannabinoid;
ECS	endocannabinoids system;
EEG	electroencephalography;
EPSP	excitatory post-synaptic potential;
FCA	fear-conditioned aversion;
F-CPA	formalin-induced conditioned place avoidance (test);
fMRI	functional magnetic resonance imaging;
FT	formalin test;
GABA	gamma amino butyric acid;
GPCR	G protein-coupled receptor;
HF	hippocampal formation;
HP	hot plate (test);
IC	insular cortex;
IP_3	inositol triphosphate;
i.p.	intraperitoneal;
KOR	kappa opioid receptor;
LA	lateral amygdala (nucleus);
LC	locus coeruleus;
LPB	lateral parabrachial nucleus;
LPI	left posterior insula;
LTD	long-term depression;
LTP	long-term potentiation;
MCC	midcingulate (division) cingulate cortex;
MOR	mu opioid receptor;
NAc	nucleus accumbens;
NSAIDs	non-steroidal anti-inflammatory drugs;
OA	osteoarthritis patients;
OR	opioid receptors;
PAG	periaqueductal gray matter;
PB	parabrachial (area);
PBN	parabrachial nucleus;
PEA	N-palmitoylethanolamide;
pERK	(protein RNA-like endoplasmic reticulum kinase);
PET	positron emission tomography;
PFC	prefrontal cortex;
PI	posterior insula;

List of Abbreviations

PIC	posterior insular cortex;
PMRS	proton magnetic resonance spectroscopy;
PSI	posterior superior insula;
PV	parvalbumin (neurons);
rMANOVA	repeated measure analysis of variance;
s.c.	subcutaneous;
RVM	rostral ventro-medial (medulla);
SI/SII	primary/secondary somatosensory cortex;
SNI	spared nerve injury;
SPA	spino-parabrachial-amygdalar (pathway);
STC	spino-thalamo-cortical (pathway);
TF	tail flick (test)
THC	Δ^{-9}-tetrahydrocannabinol;
TRP	transient receptor potential (channels);
VIP	vasoactive intestinal peptide;
VTA	ventral tegmental area;
2-AG	2-arachidonoylglycerol.

Chapter 1

INTRODUCTION

The ability to detect noxious stimuli is essential to an organism's survival and wellbeing. The nervous system by special receptors detects and interprets a wide range of environmental and endogenous stimuli, as well as varied mechanical, thermal and chemical irritants. When intense, these stimuli activate pain receptors (nociceptors) generating acute pain, and in the setting of persistent injury, both peripheral and central nervous system (CNS) components of the pain transmission pathway exhibit tremendous plasticity, enhancing pain signals and producing hypersensitivity. These mechanisms are an important component of the protective system and permanent regulator of homeostatic reaction of the body (Apkarian, 2019; Bannister et al., 2017; Basbaum et al., 2009; Da Silva et al., 2019; Seymur, Dolan, 2013).

While acute pain states generally resolve in most patients, chronic pain is an important public health problem and represents an urgent medical need worldwide. Chronic or severe pain negatively impacts quality of life of affected individuals driving patients to seek medical attention, and exacts an enormous socio-economic cost (Ossipov et al., 2014).

Classically, pain has been conceptualized from the narrow viewpoint of nociceptive processing (Baliki, Apkarian, 2015). In 1906 Charles Sherrington coined the term nociception (latin *nocere* 'to harm or hurt') and outlined its underlying neural structures. He viewed nociceptive reflexes and pain perception as tightly linked processes of transduction, transmission, and spinal cord processing of noxious signals related to primary afferents, their spinal cord circuitry, and related specialized pathways in the brain that mediate pain-like behavior (Apkarian, 2019).

On the other hand, modern neuroimaging approaches have been used to examine pain-related brain activity as a physiological biomarker of pain for treatment development (Bingel, Tracey, 2008; Bushnell et al., 2013; Da Silva et al., 2019; Kuner, Flor, 2017). Though the challenge of pain biomarker development is increased when chronic pain conditions are analyzed, a growing body of work examining the neural correlates of experimentally-induced, nociceptive pain in healthy volunteers has led to important insights into the mechanisms and characteristics of how the sensation of pain arises, including its cognitive, affective, and sensory dimensions. The functional magnetic resonance imaging (fMRI) analyses have identified several brain regions that are engaged under pain conditions, including the primary and secondary somatosensory cortex (SI/SII), insula, cingulate cortex, thalamus and somewhat less reliable, periaqueductal gray matter (PAG) and other brain structures (Bingel, Tracey, 2008; Bushnell et al., 2013; Kuner, Flor, 2017; Xu et al., 2020).

Brain limbic system, firstly described by Papez (1937) and then expanded by MacLean (1952), mostly the anterior cingulate cortex (ACC), insula and amygdala, is involved in affective aspects of pain and regulate emotional and motivational responses. These brain areas are not activated separately; they are functionally connected and contribute in a combined fashion to pain processing (Yang, Chang, 2019). Changes in emotional and motivational cues can affect the intensity and degree of pain experience (Bushnell et al., 2013; Cai et al., 2018; Leknes, Tracey, 2008; Kuner, Flor, 2017; Morris et al., 2018).

The role of opioids in the treatment of pain has been long known for the humankind for thousands of years (Tsagareli, 2012, 2018). Opioid analgesics are widely to relief dull, poorly localized (usually, visceral) pain, and especially cancer pain (Azzam et al., 2019; Ballantyne, Sullivan. 2017; Dickenson, Kieffer, 2013; Petzke et al., 2020; Schmidt et al, 2010). Repeated doses may cause tolerance to these drugs and dependence, and so that the sudden termination of opioid analgesics may precipitate a withdrawal syndrome. Apart from the opioid drugs, non-opioid, non-steroidal anti-inflammatory drugs (NSAIDs) are the most widely used analgesics in the treatment of mild or moderate pain. These drugs have analgesic, antipyretic, and at higher doses, anti-inflammatory actions. Aspirin (acetylsalicylic acid) was the first NSAID but has been largely replaced by drugs that are less toxic to gastro-intestinal tract, e.g., paracetamol, ibuprofen, ketorolac, naproxen, lornoxicam and others. NSAIDs produce their effects by inhibiting cyclo-oxygenase (COX), a key enzyme in the production of prostaglandins. The latter are one of the mediators released at sites of inflammation. They do not themselves cause pain but they potentiate the pain caused by other mediators, e.g., bradykinin, histamine, serotonin (Tsagareli, Tsiklauri, 2012; Zeilhofer, Brune, 2013; Vuilleumier et al., 2018).

Non-opioid analgesics elicit antinociception by action on the CNS structures, besides their well-known action on peripheral tissues. The analgesic effects of non-opioid drugs are due to their action on three major sites, namely, peripheral inflamed tissues, spinal cord, and the brain stem. At the latter level, non-opioid analgesics induce antinociception probably by activation of the PAG and the rostral ventro-medial part of medulla (RVM). They are considered as a descending pain control or modulatory system, which inhibits transmission of pain signals at the spinal dorsal horn. This descending modulatory circuit is an "opioid-sensitive" and relevant to human experience in many settings, including in states of chronic pain, and in the actions of pain-relieving drugs, including opiates, cannabinoids, NSAIDs, and serotonin/ norepinephrine reuptake blockers that mimic, in part, the actions of opiates (Bingel, Tracey, 2008; Heinricher, Fields, 2013; Heinricher, Ingram, 2009; Hemington, Coulombe, 2015; Ossipov et al, 2010; Ren, Dubner, 2009). At the same time, these structures probably play a crucial role in the development of tolerance to opioids and NSAIDs (Heinricher, Ingram, 2009; Lane et al., 2005; Macey et al., 2015; Vanegas et al., 2010; Vuilleumier et al., 2018).

Along with opioid mechanisms, the second neuro-modulatory system involved in the pathophysiology of pain that has recently raised a particular interest for the development of new therapeutic strategies is the endocannabinoids system (ECS) that plays a key role in pain control. This system is integrated by the cannabinoids receptors, their endogenous ligands, and the enzymes involved in the synthesis and degradation of these ligands (Di Marzo 2018; Di Marzo et al., 2015;

Hohmann, Rice, 2013; Lau, Vaughan, 2014; Maldonado et al., 2016). At least two different cannabinoid receptors, (CB1) and (CB2), have been identified (Guindon, Hohmann, 2008; Khasabova et al., 2011). Both receptors are seven trans-membrane domain receptors coupled to inhibitory G proteins, and their distribution and physiological role are quite different (Maldonado et al., 2016; Pertwee et al., 2010).

The principal goal of this book is to present main findings of the study of brain mechanisms of non-opioid induced antinociceptive tolerance in one of pain models of rats, such as the "formalin test". In particular, the principal purpose was to examine a relation between administration of NSAIDs in brain limbic areas, – the anterior cingulated cortex, rostral insular cortex, and central amygdala causing tolerance, – and brain endogenous antinociceptive PAG and RVM sites. By microinjection NSAIDs (diclofenac, ketoprofen, ketorolac, and lornoxicam) into the limbic cerebral structures for consecutive four days, we studied the mechanisms of responsiveness of these brain areas to tolerance induced by these drugs to the thermal and mechanical painful stimulation. Also, we tested opioid sensitivity of these brain emotional-motivational areas by injection of morphine receptors antagonists' naloxone and octapeptide CTOP (D-phe-Cys-Tyr-D-Trp-Orn-Thr-Pen-Thr-$_{NH2}$) by pre- and post-treatment to NSAIDs. CTOP is a cyclic analog of the neuropeptide somatostatin and is known to block the analgesic effect of morphine, selectively bind its mu-opioid receptor. In the other series of experiments to test ECS involvement in tolerance effects to NSAIDs, CB1 receptor antagonist AM-251 were microinjected into these brain limbic areas, and the PAG. Our hypothesis was based on the suggestion that the central antinociceptive effects of NSAIDs probably involve the endogenous opioid and cannabinoid systems of descending pain control PAG–RVM axis.

Chapter 2

BRAIN LIMBIC AREAS AND PAIN

Emotional distress is an intrinsic and the most disruptive and undesirable feature of painful states. Pain sensation is characterized as a complex experience, dependent not only on the regulation of nociceptive sensory systems (a sensory-discriminative component) but also on the activation of mechanisms that control emotional processes (an emotional-motivational component) in brain limbic areas such as the hypothalamus, amygdala, and hippocampus (Craig, 2006; Keay, Bandler, 2009; Seymur, Dolan, 2013). First classic experiments in Melzack's laboratory by injection of local anesthetics into limbic structures – such as the lateral hypothalamus, the cingulum and the hippocampal formation – showed a temporary block of neural activity and an induction of significant analgesia during late tonic phase of pain perception (Tasker et al., 1987; Vaccarino, Melzack, 1989; McKena, Melzack, 1992). The involvement of hippocampal formation including dorsal hippocampus (DH) in nociception and some abnormalities in hippocampal functioning with persistent pain have been shown later (Favaroni Mendes, Menescal-de-Oliveira, 2008; Liu, Chen, 2009; Mutzo et al., 2012). Furthermore, surgical lesions of the cingulate cortex and/or the cingulum bundle reduced the emotional but not the sensory component of chronic pain (Corkin, Hebben, 1981). On the basis one of the first positron emission tomography (PET) studies, it has been concluded that activation of structures associated with autonomic and limbic system functions, such as the insula and the ACC, may reflect the affective aspect of pain experience (Casey, 2000).

A network analysis suggested that there are broad-ranging, as well as specific, changes that are related to various chronic pain syndromes, with a focus on prefrontal regions, the anterior insula, ACC, basal ganglia, thalamus, PAG, post- and pre-central gyri and inferior parietal lobule (Kuner, Flor, 2017). (Figure 1). Despite several commonalities, chronic pain syndromes of different etiologies can be mechanistically distinct and show different clinical manifestations. Chronic inflammatory and muscular pain disorders involve a constant ongoing stream of nociceptive inputs from the affected tissues to peripheral and central nociceptive pathways (Kuner, Flor, 2017).

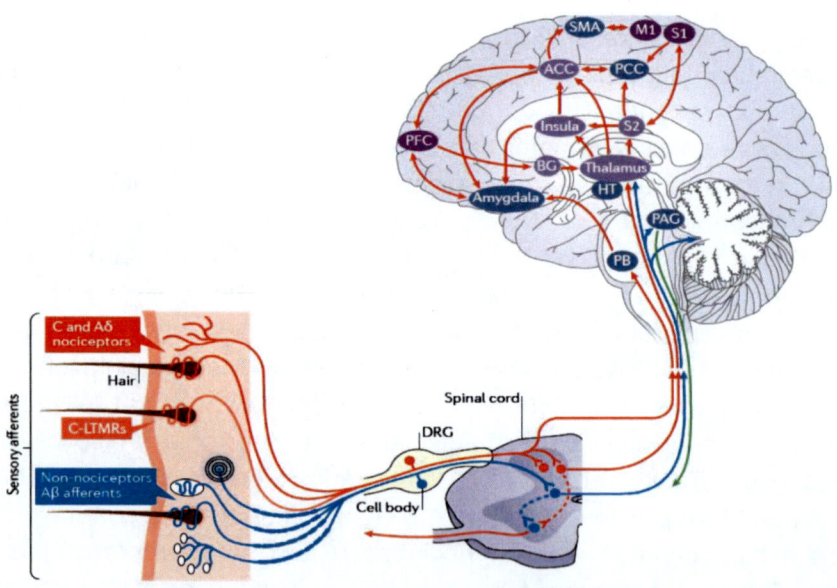

Figure 1. Nociceptive pathways from peripheral receptors through the spinal cord to pain-related brain regions. A red line–spino-midbrain-forebrain pathways; a blue line–spino-mesencephalic and spino-cerebellar pathways; a green line–a midbrain descending pathway. Abbreviations: ACC, anterior cingulate cortex; BG, basal ganglia; HT, hypothalamus; M1, primary motor cortex; PAG, periaqueductal grey; PB, parabrachial nucleus; PCC, posterior cingulate cortex; PFC, prefrontal cortex; S1, primary somatosensory cortex; SMA, supplementary motor area; C-LTMRs, C–low-threshold mechano-receptors (Adapted from Kuner, Flor, 2017, with permission).

At the same time, chronic pain represents a complex disorder with anxio-depressive symptoms and cognitive deficits. Underlying mechanisms are still not well understood but an important role for interactions between prefrontal cortical areas and subcortical limbic structures has emerged evidence from preclinical studies in the rodent brain suggests that neuroplastic changes in prefrontal (anterior cingulate, prelimbic and infralimbic) cortical and subcortical (amygdala and nucleus accumbens) brain areas and their interactions (cortico-limbic circuitry) contribute to the complexity and persistence of pain and may be predetermining factors has been proposed in recent human neuroimaging studies and meta-analysis (Henssen et al., 2019; Thompson, Neugebauer, 2019; Volkers et al., 2020; Xu et al., 2020).

Chronic neuropathic pain, in this regard, is associated with an imbalance of activity in pathways that results from loss or interruption of physiological inputs due to lesions to peripheral or central neurons. Several clinical pain disorders involve inflammatory and neuropathic components. A large body of converging evidence suggests that chronic pain is not simply a temporal extension of acute pain but involves distinct mechanisms. The transition of acute pain into a chronic disorder involves activity-dependent functional plastic changes or sensitization at many different inter-connected levels, ranging from the molecular to the network level, at several anatomical avenues in the nociceptive pathway (Prescott et al., 2014).

Mechanisms involving functional plasticity have been studied extensively and have revealed a range of modulatory factors that change the sensory, emotional and cognitive components of pain (Apkarian et al., 2009; Basbaum et al., 2009). However, recent data show that functional plasticity changes are accompanied by structural remodeling and reorganization of synapses, cells and circuits that can also occur at various anatomical and temporal scales, thereby further adding complexity and a large dynamic range, and potentially accounting for the development of pain that extends over longer periods of time (Figure 2). Structural remodeling of connections has not been studied as widely as functional plasticity, and it remains unclear whether it represents a cause or a consequence of chronic pain (Kuner, Flor, 2017).

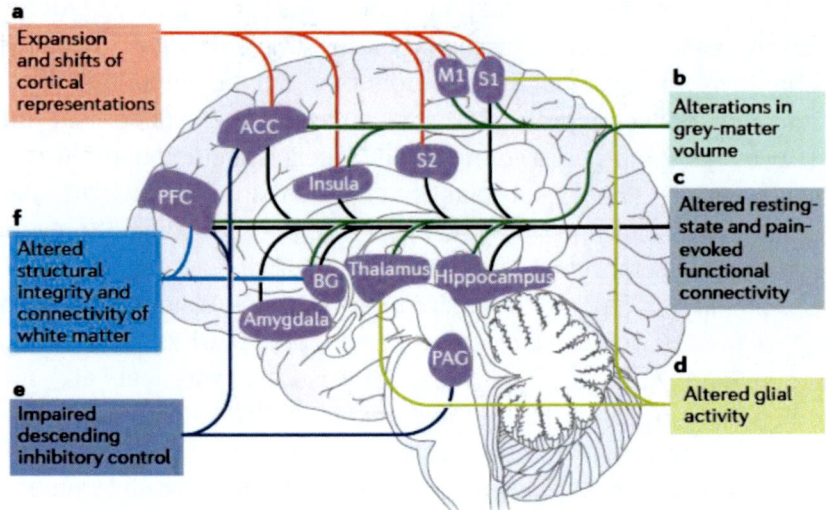

Figure 2. Structural and functional changes in the human different brain areas in chronic pain conditions. Abbreviations: ACC, anterior cingulate cortex; BG, basal ganglia; M1, primary motor cortex; PAG, periaqueductal grey; PFC, prefrontal cortex; S1, primary somatosensory cortex; S2, secondary somatosensory cortex. (Reproduced from Kuner, Flor, 2017, with permission).

ANTERIOR CINGULATE CORTEX

As stated above, pain is a complex experience involving sensory, motivational and cognitive components. Such diversity is supported by a variety of ascending pathways conveying nociceptive information from the spinal cord to the forebrain, of which the two main routes are the spino-thalamo-cortical (STC) and the spino-parabrachial-amygdalar (SPA) tracts. After relay in multiple nuclei of the posterior thalamus, the STC pathway in primates, targets three main cortical regions involved in sensorimotor integration and attentional drive, namely the posterior insula, the medial parietal operculum, and the mid-cingulate cortex. The spino-parabrachial route, on the other hand, reaches the limbic system *via* the amygdalar complex, especially its central nucleus, and participates to the triggering of autonomic responses and the elaboration of affective components of pain (Bastuji et al., 2018).

The ACC is a part of the brain limbic system, and located in the frontal part of the cingulate cortex in the inner side of the cerebral hemispheres. The ACC is a complex and heterogeneous cortex, receives afferent inputs mainly from the medial thalamic nuclei (midline and intra-laminar nuclei) that contain nociceptive neurons receiving inputs from the spino-thalamic tract. The involvement of the ACC in pain perception is based on its extensive afferent projections from the medio-dorsal thalamic nucleus and widespread inter-connections with relevant regions of the descending pain modulation system. A projection from the spinal dorsal horn through the medial/intra-laminar thalamic nuclei to the ACC has been proposed to process information on pain-related unpleasantness (Xiao, Zhang, 2018).

In addition, to contributing to the immediate affective consequences of noxious stimulation, the ACC may contribute to avoidance learning. Neurons in the rostral ACC (rACC) are required for pain-related aversive learning – a process that directly reflects the affective component of pain (Johansen et al., 2001). This group of scholars further found that the activation of rACC, but not caudal ACC neurons is necessary and sufficient to encode pain-related aversive emotions. Intra-ACC injections of an excitatory amino acid antagonist blocked the formalin-induced conditioned place aversion (F-CPA) acquisition rather than formalin-induced acute inflammatory pain, indicating that the reduction of pain-related aversion is not due to a general decrease in the nociceptive processing of inflammatory pain (Johansen, Fields, 2004). Consistent with this, proton magnetic resonance spectroscopy (PMRS) has revealed an altered metabolite status in the ACC of chronic pain patients compared to controls. The mean levels of glutamic acid (Glu)/total creatine and Glu + glutamine/total creatine are higher, but lower for N-acetyl-aspartate/total creatine, in the chronic pain patients, concluding that they have a different, some higher metabolite status in the ACC to healthy controls (Ito et al., 2017).

It is interesting that as pain is aversive reaction its relief elicits reward mediated by dopaminergic signaling in the nucleus accumbens (NAc). Endogenous opioid signaling in the ACC, an area encoding pain aversiveness, contributes to pain modulation. It has been found that endogenous ACC opioid neurotransmission is required for relief of pain and subsequent downstream activation of dopamine signaling

(Navratilova et al., 2015). These authors provide a neural explanation for the preferential effects of opioids on pain affect and demonstrate that engagement of NAc dopaminergic transmission by non-opioid pain-relieving treatments depends on upstream ACC opioid circuits. Thus, endogenous opioid signaling in the ACC appears to be both necessary and sufficient for relief of pain aversiveness (Navratilova et al., 2015). Furthermore, this group of researchers has just demonstrated that engagement of mu-opioid receptors in the right central nucleus of amygdala (CeA) modulates affective qualities of ongoing pain through endogenous opioid neurotransmission within the rACC, revealing opioid-dependent functional connections from the CeA to the rACC, and hence resulting in enhancement of net descending inhibition (Navratilova et al., 2020).

There are increasing studies from both animal and human investigations that demonstrate the importance of the ACC and IC as well as prefrontal cortex (PFC) and primary and secondary somatosensory cortices (SI/SII) in chronic pain and related emotional disorders in different models of chronic pain. In particular for the ACC and IC, hyper-excitation or hyper-activation has been observed in different chronic pain conditions. This observation in humans has also been confirmed by animal studies that neurons in these cortical areas respond to peripheral noxious stimuli or injury. For example, in adult rats, peripheral amputation caused long-term potentiation (LTP) in the *in vivo* ACC (Zhuo, 2016a, 2019).

It has recently been shown that the midcingulate division of the cingulate cortex (MCC) does not mediate acute pain sensation and pain affect, but gates sensory hypersensitivity by acting in a wide cortical and subcortical network. Within this complex network, an afferent MCC–PI (posterior insula) pathway can induce and maintain nociceptive hypersensitivity in the absence of conditioned peripheral noxious drive. This facilitation of nociception is brought about by recruitment of descending serotoninergic (*via* the nucleus raphe magnus) facilitatory projections to the spinal cord dorsal horn. These results have implications for further understanding of neuronal mechanisms facilitating the transition from acute to chronic, long-lasting pain (Tan et al., 2017).

INSULAR CORTEX

The insula nicely demonstrates the convergence of neuroanatomy and the multidimensional nature of pain. This phylogenetically ancient structure appears to receive information *via* a direct thalamo-insular connection and can be thought of as a site for sensory and affective integration (Bastuji, et al., 2018; Benarroch et al., 2019; Craig, 2006; Brooks, Tracey, 2007; Henderson et al., 2007).

Cytoarchitectonically, the insular cortex is a complex and richly connected structure that functions as a cortical hub involved in interoception, multimodal sensory processing, autonomic control, perceptual self-awareness, and emotional guidance of social behavior. The human insula is subdivided into a posterior and an anterior lobe and includes posterior, middle, and anterior subdivisions based on different cytoarchitectonics (granular, dysgranular, and agranular), connectivity, and functions. The posterior (granular) insula receives inputs from pain, temperature, visceral, vestibular, and other sensory pathways; this multimodal sensory representation is further elaborated in the mid-insular (dysgranular) cortex and then conveyed to the anterior (agranular) insula, which further processes this information and interacts with areas involved in cognitive and emotional control. The insula thus provides an interface between bodily sensation, pain, and emotion, and may have a key role in perceptual awareness, social behavior, and decision making (Benarroch, 2019).

A growing body of literature suggests that the brain region that is a part of the pain processing network, the insula, is both anatomically and functionally well suited to serve a primary and fundamental role in pain processing (Amanzio, Palermo, 2019; Benarroch, 2019; Lu et al., 2016; Nieuwenhuys, 2012; Tsiklauri et al., 2018). By quantitative perfusion neuroimaging to investigate slowly varying neural states highly relevant to a complex phenomenon, such as pain, a group of Irene Tracey identified the dorsal posterior insula as sub-serving a fundamental role in pain and the likely human homolog of the nociceptive region identified from animal studies (Segerdahl et al, 2015). Especially with regard to pain experience, the insular cortex (IC) has been supposed to participate in both sensory-discriminative and affective-motivational aspects of pain (Lu et al., 2016). In the course of pain anticipation, neural activations were discovered by fMRI in the dorsolateral prefrontal, mid-cingulate, and anterior insula cortices; medial and inferior frontal gyri; inferior parietal lobule; middle and superior temporal gyri, and thalamus and caudate nucleus as well (Amanzio, Palermo, 2019; Palermo et al., 2015).

Very interesting data were obtained by depth stereotactic electroencephalography (EEG) exploration of the IC for pre-surgical evaluation in 142 epilepsy patients undergoing insular electrical stimulations. The authors found a somatotopic organization of sites where stimulation produced pain and that was observed along the rostro-caudal and vertical axis of the insula, showing a face representation rostral to those of upper and lower limbs, with an upper limb representation located above that of the lower limb (Mazzola et al., 2009). They suggested that, in spite of large and often bilateral receptive fields, pain representation shows some degree of somatotopic organization in the human insula (Mazzola et al., 2009).

The anterior or agranular insular cortex (AIC) is found in other mammals including cats, monkeys, and primates including humans. In primates, the divisions of the IC are the same as in rats and the AIC occupies an area immediately noticeable, that is, dorsal to the primary olfactory cortex. The rat's AIC is a small region of the cerebral cortex located on the lateral area of the cerebral hemispheres that is involved in the perception and response to pain (Jasmin, Ohara, 2009). Direct injections of morphine into the AIC increasing dopamine and gamma amino butyric acid (GABA) levels result in behavioral antinociception (Jasmin et al., 2003). The major connections of the AIC are with areas that have established roles in behavior responses to nociceptive stimuli. The AIC projections to other cortical areas and subcortical sites such as the amygdala are likely to participate in the sensorimotor integration of nociceptive processing, while the hypothalamus and brainstem projections are most likely to contribute to descending pain inhibitory control (Jasmin, Ohara, 2009).

The human posterior insula is able to encode sensory aspects of nociceptive input including intensity, somatotopy and sensory sub-modality (Bastuji et al., 2018). Intracranial laser evoked potential recordings suggest a rapid information flow from posterior to anterior insula, – the latter being an agranular cortex implicated in integrative aspects of pain, including affective and visceral reactions associated to the painful sensation. The connectivity patterns of posterior and anterior insula differ substantially. The anterior portions of the insula, together with the temporal pole and lateral orbito-frontal cortex, were termed *"paralimbic"* because of their extensive reciprocal inter-connections with limbic structures in rhesus monkeys (Bastuji et al., 2018). Human experiments analyzing nociceptive-specific evoked potentials and functional connectivity in ten epileptic patients with electrodes simultaneously implanted in the posterior and anterior insular sectors, as well as in the amygdala nucleus showed exceptional access to responses in the three regions allowed analyzing both response timing and functional inter-areal relationships *via* phase-coherence, and generated a comprehensive image of the activities of the three structures. The results suggest that, during the first second that follows a noxious stimulus, an initial parallel and uncorrelated nociceptive processing in sensory and limbic systems is rapidly followed by a functional convergence of both toward the anterior insula (Bastuji et al., 2018). The results point to the anterior insula as an area of sensory-limbic convergence, integrating sensory with emotional input, and hence participating in the transformation of cortical nociception into the experience of pain (Bastuji et al., 2018).

As stated above, along with the ACC, Zhuo and his group found that IC, the second principal cortical area for pain, is highly plastic and can undergo LTP after injury. Inhibiting IC LTP reduces behavioral sensitization caused by injury. LTP of glutamatergic transmission in pain-related cortical areas serves as a key mechanism for developing chronic pain (Liu et al., 2013; Zhuo, 2016b, 2019).

ANTERIOR CINGULATE AND INSULAR CORTICES: TWO FUNCTIONALLY CONNECTED AREAS FOR PAIN

Among several cortical regions of the cerebrum, IC and ACC are two common brain areas that are activated by pain processing (Apkarian et al., 2005; Bushnell et al., 2013). The IC receives afferent projections from thalamic nuclei, and it forms reciprocal connections with the ACC, amygdala, limbic system, and cortical association areas (Figure 3).

These anatomic connections provide the basis for its important roles in pain perception (Craig, 2006, 2014; Jasmin, Ohara, 2009).

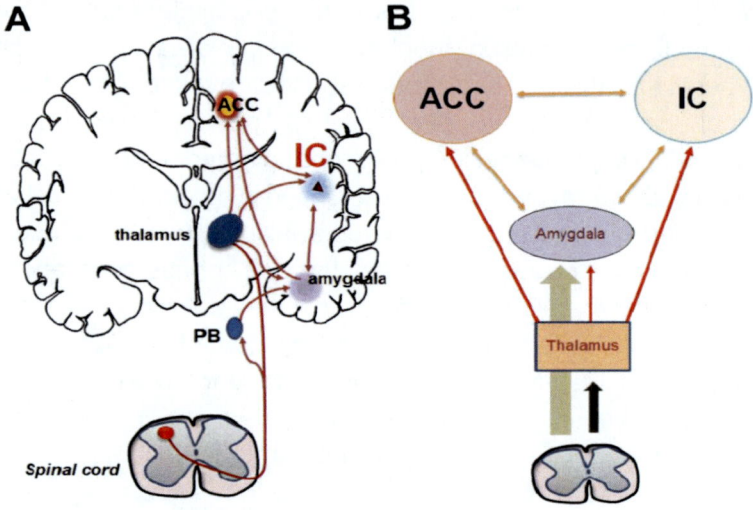

Figure 3. Models for the IC in pain transmission and chronic pain. (A) A simplified diagram shows that IC receives sensory nociceptive information from the spinal cord, through the thalamus and amygdala. It also forms interaction with neurons in the ACC. (B) A model for two critical cortical regions, ACC and IC in pain. Neurons in the ACC and IC have been reported to be involved in pain perception, including unpleasantness in chronic pain conditions. They receive nociceptive or unpleasant emotional information through thalamus and amygdala. The interaction between ACC/IC and amygdala are bi-directional and providing possible reinforcement as well as compensatory mechanisms at subcortical and cortical levels. Abbreviations: ACC, anterior cingulate cortex; IC, insular cortex; PB, parabrachial area (Reproduced from Zhuo, 2016b, with permission).

It is clear that both ACC and IC may contribute to the central process of painful information. The anatomic evidence suggests that neurons in ACC and IC are likely interacted. Furthermore, both ACC and IC form bi-redirectional projections with neurons in the amygdala. Such cortical and subcortical circuits provide reliable foundation for animals and human to process unpleasant and/or fearful information. In pathological conditions, they also contribute to long-term suffering of these patients emotionally such as long-term anxiety and depression caused chronic pain disease. Inhibiting injury-related plasticity in both cortical areas may give better opportunities to control chronic pain (Zhuo, 2016b).

It has recently been analyzed the effect of a learned increase in the dissociation between the rACC and the left posterior insula (LPI) on pain intensity and unpleasantness, and the contribution of each region to the effect, exploring the possibility to influence the perception of pain with neuro-feedback methods (Rance et al, 2014). They found by fMRI study in ten subjects trained on four consecutive days that subjects were able to increase the difference in all four conditions after six training trials, thus successfully achieving the two states of either the rACC or the LPI of the blood oxygenation level-dependent (BOLD) percent signal change being higher. When looking at the contribution of the single regions to the combined difference feedback, the LPI was found to be driving force in three out of the four conditions with significant changes in the activation from the first to the last training trial. Activation in the rACC did not change significantly. These results suggested that in the modulation of pain intensity and unpleasantness, both the rACC and LPI either alone or combined, did not sufficient to alter perception of the painful experimental electric stimulus. However, it is possible that increasing automatization of the response would free the respective region from dual tasking and could thus have an effect (Rance et al, 2014).

The rACC is distinct from the subdivisions of mid-cingulate cortex (MCC) and the posterior cingulate cortex in the dorsal and caudal ACC, respectively. How this anatomical diversity is translated into functional differences has not been considered in pain and may underlie the diverse putative functions described for the cingulate cortex in pain modulation. Recently it has reported that activation of MCC–to–PI (posterior insula) afferents alone can generate a state of nociceptive hypersensitivity independent of a peripheral nociceptive conditioning input. This has implications for changes in pain sensitivity reported in patients in the absence of (or persisting following healing of) obvious injuries or physical pathologies. These data provide a mechanistic basis for exacerbation of pain by psychosocial factors that may deregulate basal activity in the MCC and the PI; and thus, give insights into cortical circuitry involved in the transition from acute to persistent pain (Tan et al., 2017).

This comprehensive study reveals a pathway from the MCC to the PI that is sufficient to induce and maintain nociceptive hypersensitivity even in the absence of nociceptive drive. This pathway interacts with descending pain modulatory systems located in the raphe nuclei. Functionally, the MCC modulates pain independently of the emotional or affective dimension of pain that is controlled by the rACC (Figure 4).

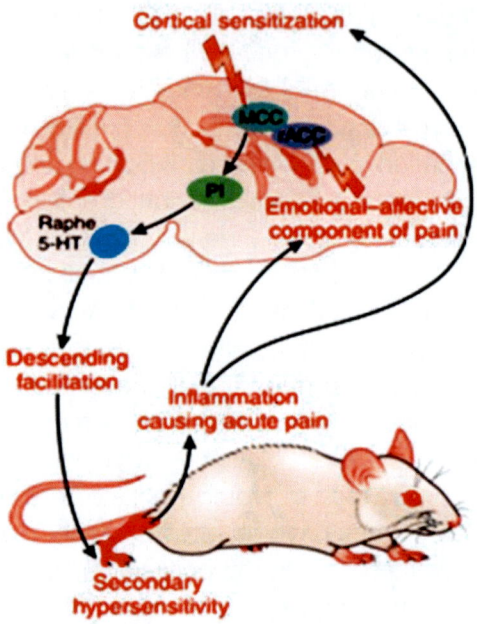

Figure 4. Cortical sensitization gates sensory hypersensitivity. Increased noxious drive (i.e., during inflammation, produced here by nearby injection of capsaicin into hindpaw) results in long-lasting cortical sensitization in the MCC that controls a network involving the posterior insular cortex (PI) and the serotoninergic raphe nuclei. This pathway induces and maintains secondary hypersensitivity that transits acute into chronic pain. (Reproduced from Nevian, 2017, with permission).

This newly identified afferent pathway from the MCC to the posterior insula that induces and maintains nociceptive hypersensitivity needs more attention in future research. It will be of great interest to unravel the underlying circuit and cellular plasticity mechanisms that cause the sensitized state. This insight may suggest ways to prevent the induction of hypersensitivity or reverse this chronic state once it is induced. Since this seminal finding yields insight into the transition from acute to chronic pain, the revelation of the underlying mechanisms will have high translational potential. But beyond that, this study shows that cortical brain regions strongly influence spinal pain processing *via* the descending neuromodulatory system (Nevian, 2017).

CENTRAL NUCLEUS OF AMYGDALA

The amygdala has emerged as a key brain region that modulates aversive responses to pain, fear and stress (Baliki, Apkarian, 2015; Neugebauer, 2015). Neuroimaging studies have demonstrated that amygdala function and connectivity are altered in patients with chronic pain, suggesting that amygdala hypersensitivity may contribute to chronic or persistent pain (Bingel, Tracey, 2008; Bushnell et al., 2013; Kuner, Flor, 2017). However, neural mechanisms underlying amygdala sensitization are not well understood (Navratilova et al., 2019; 2020).

The amygdala as an important component of the limbic system participates in the control of the pain response and modulates the affective-motivational aspect of pain. The central nucleus (CeA), basolateral (BLA) and lateral (LA) nuclei of the amygdala are involved in the processing and regulation of chronic pain. The anterior and posterior portions of the BLA and the central portion of the CeA are involved in controlling neuropathic pain. The inactivation of these nuclei reversed hyperalgesia, allodynia and depressive-like behavior in animals with peripheral neuropathy. These findings confirm the neuro-circuitry involved in persistent pain and the roles of specific amygdala subnuclei in the modulation of neuropathic pain, including the neurocircuitry that processes the affective-motivational component of pain (Seno et al., 2018).

Concerning the interconnections of the several functionally and structurally distinct nuclei that amygdala encompasses with other brain areas, the lateral subdivision of the CeA receives direct nociceptive input from calcitonin gene-related peptide (CGRP)-expressing neurons in the parabrachial area (PB) as well as contextual pain information from the cortex and lateral–basolateral amygdala. The CeA contains mostly gamma amino-butyric acid neurons, some of which also co-express neuropeptides such as corticotrophin-releasing factor (CRF) and dynorphin, an endogenous agonist at kappa opioid receptors (KORs). Direct projections from CeA CRF neurons to brainstem areas including the PB and the PAG promote aversive and anxiety-like behaviors (Navratilova et al., 2019). This group of scholars has found that KOR circuits in the undergo neuroplasticity in chronic neuropathic pain resulting in increased sensory and affective pain responses, and thus KOR antagonists may therefore represent novel therapies for neuropathic pain by targeting aversive aspects of ongoing pain while preserving protective functions of acute pain (Navratilova et al., 2019).

In the other study has been shown that activation of the excitatory pathway from the parabrachial nucleus (PBN) that relays peripheral pain signals to the CeA is sufficient to cause behaviors of negative emotions including anxiety, depression, and aversion in normal rats. In strong contrast, activation of the excitatory pathway from BLA that conveys processed cortico-limbic signals to CeA dramatically opposes these behaviors of negative emotion, reducing anxiety and depression, and induces behavior of reward. Surprisingly, activating the PBN – CeA pathway to simulate pain signals does not change pain sensitivity itself, but activating the BLA – CeA pathway inhibits basal and sensitized pain (Cai et al., 2018). These findings demonstrate that the pain signal conveyed through the PBN – CeA pathway is sufficient to drive negative emotion and that the cortico-limbic signal *via* the BLA – CeA pathway counteracts the negative emotion, suggesting a top-down brain mechanism for cognitive control of negative emotion under stressful environmental conditions such as pain (Cai et al., 2018).

In this regard, mice expressing fear-conditioned analgesia (FCA) displayed an increase in c-Fos/CaMKII (Ca^{2+}/calmodulin-dependent protein kinase II) co-localization in the lateral amygdala and BLA compared to controls. Additionally, a significant increase in cFos/CRF co-localization was observed in mice expressing FCA. These results show that amygdala processing of conditioned contextual aversive, nociceptive, and FCA behaviors involve different neuronal phenotypes and neural circuits between, within, and from various amygdala nuclei. In particular, the BLA contains (CaMKII) and parvalbumin (PV) neurons; the CeA neurons are primarily inhibitory (GABA-ergic) that comprise enkephalin interneurons and CRF neurons that project to the PAG. This information will be important in developing novel therapies for treating pain and emotive disorders in humans (Butler et al., 2017). On the other hand, it has just been found that glutamate A1 (GluA1) receptors in the

CeA promote opioid use and its upregulation is sufficient to increase opioid consumption, which counteracts the acute inhibitory effect of pain on opioid intake. These results demonstrate that the CeA GluA1 is a shared target of opioid and pain in regulation of opioid use, which may aid in future development of therapeutic applications in opioid abuse (Hou et al., 2020).

Recently, an interesting model on neural mechanisms underlying bidirectional modulation of pain was proposed demonstrating that the CeA functions as a pain rheostat, decreasing or increasing pain-related behaviors in mice. This dual and opposing function of the CeA is encoded by opposing changes in the excitability of two distinct subpopulations of GABA-ergic neurons that receive excitatory inputs from the PBN. Thus, cells expressing protein kinase C-delta (CeA-PKCd) are sensitized by nerve injury and increase pain-related responses. In contrast, cells expressing somatostatin (CeA-Som) are inhibited by nerve injury and their activity drives antinociception. These results demonstrate that the CeA can amplify or suppress pain in a cell-type-specific manner, uncovering a previously unknown mechanism underlying bidirectional control of pain in the brain (Wilson et al., 2019).

HIPPOCAMPUS AND PAIN

The hippocampus, a part of the limbic system, has the function of learning and memory, emotion and affect, and also has relationships with chronic and acute pain. It has been reported that hippocampal formation (HF) plays an important role in pain information processing, including anatomical features, behavioral experiments, functional imaging, electrophysiology, and other molecular research (Fasick et al., 2015; Liu, Chen, 2009; Mutso et al., 2012; McCrae et al., 2015; Wang et al., 2016).

Whereas several supra-spinal regions, including the locus coeruleus (LC) (adrenergic neuron cell bodies), hippocampus (contains adrenergic nerve terminals extending from the LC), PAG, and RVM play a key role in modulating pain signals; brain regions such as the PFC, ACC, thalamus, and hippocampus are activated during pain processing (Apkarian et al., 2005). The hippocampus participates in both the processing and modification of nociceptive stimuli. Several experimental studies have found that direct manipulation of the hippocampus alters nociceptive behavior. Injection of lidocaine, a local anesthetic with sodium channel-blocking effect, directly into the dentate gyrus produces analgesia (McEwen, 2001; McKenna, Melzack, 1992). Stimulation of the dorsal hippocampus (DH) affects nociception without being aversive, supporting the hippocampal contribution to pain awareness (Lathe, 2001). Furthermore, a lesion in the hippocampus can alter the perception of noxious stimuli and partially alleviate pain (Al Amin et al., 2004; Maletic et al., 2007). The hippocampus can also be altered by peripheral manipulation. In an animal model of chronic inflammatory pain, a unilateral, hindpaw injection of complete Freund's adjuvant caused bilateral neuro-degeneration in the hippocampus (Duric, McCarson, 2005, 2007). All these observations support the notion that the hippocampus is involved in the development and reoccurring effects of chronic pain (Fasick et al., 2015).

Similar to these data it has been found that spared nerve injury (SNI) neuropathic pain in mice was unable to extinguish contextual fear and showed increased anxiety-like behavior. Additionally, SNI mice compared with sham animals exhibited hippocampal (1) reduced extracellular signal-regulated kinase expression and phosphorylation, (2) decreased neurogenesis, and (3) altered short-term synaptic plasticity. To relate the observed hippocampal abnormalities with human chronic pain, the volume of human hippocampus in chronic back pain (CBP), complex regional pain syndrome (CRPS), and osteoarthritis patients (OA) were measured. Compared with controls, CBP and CRPS, but not OA, had significantly less bilateral hippocampal volume (Mutso et al., 2012). These results indicate that hippocampus-mediated behavior, synaptic plasticity, and neurogenesis are abnormal in neuropathic rodents. The changes may be related to the reduction in hippocampal volume that is seen in chronic pain patients, and these abnormalities may underlie learning and emotional deficits commonly observed in such patients. Therefore, targeting the reversal of these systematic changes in chronic pain could improve both patient quality of life and actual pain behavior (Mutso et al., 2012).

Other MRI study has shown that potential mechanisms for reduced hippocampal volume in fibromyalgia include abnormal glutamate excitatory neurotransmission and glucocorticoid dysfunction; these factors can lead to neuronal atrophy, through excitotoxicity, and disrupt neurogenesis in the hippocampus. Such hippocampal atrophy may play a role in memory and cognitive complaints among fibromyalgia patients (McCrae et al., 2015).

Different neurotransmitters involved in nociception are widely presented in the DH. Acetylcholine is one of the main neurotransmitters released in the DH and plays an important role in hippocampal nociceptive processing. Besides acetylcholine, evidence is accumulating that opioid peptides are important modulators of information processing in the hippocampus. When activated, opioid receptors play a key role in central pain modulation mechanisms and the hippocampal formation (HF) is a structure that expresses significant densities of this kind of receptors. The excitatory effects of opioids, including morphine, on hippocampal pyramidal cells are believed to be due to a reduction of a GABA-mediated synaptic inhibitory transmission (i.e., dis-inhibition) between interneurons and pyramidal cells in the hippocampus. Within this context, a complex interaction among these three neurotransmitter systems, cholinergic, opioidergic and GABA-ergic, seems to be involved in the modulation of the antinociceptive response. In this way, it has been demonstrated that the activation of the cholinergic or opioidergic system of the DH promotes antinociception in guinea pigs, while GABA-ergic activation promotes pro-nociception, as demonstrated by respective decreases and increases of the vocalization index. In addition, antinociception produced by cholinergic stimulation of the DH depends on opioid synapses present at the same site. On the other hand, antinociception observed after microinjection of morphine into the DH occurs through the inhibition of tonically active GABA-ergic interneurons (Favaroni Mendes, Menescal-de-Oliveira, 2008).

As stated above, the ACC and IC are involved in the contribution of plastic synaptic changes to painful information. Spatiotemporal plasticity of synaptic connection and function in the HF in response to persistent nociception is observed. In particular, peripheral strong noxious stimulation produced great impact upon the higher brain structures that lead to not only temporal plasticity, but also spatial plasticity of synaptic connection and function in the HF. The spatial plasticity of synaptic activities is more complex than the temporal plasticity, comprising of enlargement of synaptic connection size at network level, deformed the field excitatory postsynaptic potential (EPSP) at local circuit level and, increased synaptic efficacy at cellular level. In addition, the multi-synaptic model established in this investigation may open a new avenue for future studies of pain-related brain dysfunctions at the higher level of the pain neuromatrix (Zhao et al., 2009).

Concerning the transient receptor potential (TRP) channels role in hippocampal plasticity, Gibson and coauthors (2008) reported that vanilloid 1 subfamily (TRPV1) channel is a key mediator of synaptic plasticity in the hippocampus, raising intriguing questions about hippocampal function and challenging the feasibility of targeting TRPV1 for the treatment of pain. While high frequency stimulation produces LTP in pyramidal cells, it simultaneously decreases the strength of excitatory synapses from the same afferents onto inhibitory interneurons found within *stratum radiatum* (Gibson et al., 2008). This group of researchers sought to elucidate the mechanisms underlying this form of interneuron long-term depression (LTD). These results suggest that, in the hippocampus, TRPV1 receptor activation selectively modifies synapses onto interneurons (Gibson et al., 2008). Like other forms of hippocampal synaptic plasticity, TRPV1-mediated LTD may have a role in long-term changes in physiological and pathological circuit behavior during learning and epileptic activity (Alter, Gereau, 2008).

It is known that endogenous opioid peptides modulate hippocampal excitability, and the endogenous hippocampal opioid systems are implicated in learning, including that associated with drug use. The dentate gyrus (DG) contains several types of opioid peptides, which have varying degrees of receptor selectivity, and opioid receptors, which can be activated by both endogenous opioid peptides and exogenous opiate drugs (Drake et al., 2007).

Chapter 3

OPIOID AND CANNABINOID SYSTEMS

Opioids remain the drug of choice for the clinical management of moderate to severe pain. Clinical point of view, some opioids (buprenorphine, morphine, oxycodone, tramadol, tapentadol) provide substantial pain relief compared to placebo in non-cancer neuropathic pain, in particular post-herpetic neuralgia and peripheral neuropathies of different etiologies for 1-3 months. There is insufficient evidence to support or refute the suggestion that these drugs are effective in other neuropathic pain conditions. The safety of opioids with regards to abuse and deaths in the studies analyzed cannot be extrapolated to routine clinical care (Sommer et al., 2020). Similarly, within the context of randomized controlled trials of 4-15 weeks, opioids provided a clinically relevant pain relief of 30% or greater and a clinically relevant reduction of disability compared to placebo in non-malignant chronic low back pain (Petzke et al., 2020), and of in chronic osteoarthritis pain (hip, knee) for 4-24 weeks trials (Welsch et al., 2019).

However, in addition to their most effective analgesic actions, opioids also produce a sense of well-being and euphoria, which may trigger significant concerns associated with their use (Sirohi, Tiwari, 2016). The widespread abuse of prescription opioids and a dramatic increase in the availability of illicit opioids have created what is commonly referred to as the opioid epidemic. In fact, there has been an alarming increase in prescription opioid use, abuse and illicit use; and according to the National Center for Health Statistics, the total number of deaths related to opioid overdose has more than tripled from 2011 to 2014 in the USA. Increasing the availability of medication-assisted treatments (such as buprenorphine and naltrexone), the use of abuse-deterrent formulations, and the adoption of US Centers for Disease Control and Prevention (CDCP) prescribing guidelines all constitute short-term approaches to quell this epidemic, and CDCP has listed prescription opioid overdose among one of the 10 most important public health problems in all the 50 states. However, with more than 125 million Americans suffering from either acute or chronic pain, the development of effective alternatives to opioids, enabled at least in part by a fuller understanding of the neurobiological bases of pain, offers the best long-term solution for controlling and ultimately eradicating this epidemic (Skolnick, 2018).

Research over the past decade has shed light on the influence of endocannabinoids (ECs) on the opioid system. Evidence from both animal and clinical studies point toward an interaction between these two opioid and cannabinoid systems, and suggest that targeting the EC system may provide novel interventions for managing morphine addiction, opiate dependence and withdrawal reactions (Scavone et al., 2013).

OPIOID SYSTEM

The use of opium as a drug dates to thousands of years BC, and use of this extract of the exudate of *Papaver somniferum* has been traced through many ancient civilizations. Morphine, the main active agent or compound in opium, has become the *'gold standard'* analgesic to which all other opioids are compared (Dickenson, Kieffer, 2013).

Some basic analgesic drugs for systemic (intravenous, i.v., or intraperitoneal, i.p.) use were discovered in the 19th century, like as morphine, aspirin, pyramidon, paracetamol. In 1806, F.W. Sertürner reported on his discovery of the sleep-inducing substance extraction contained in opium. Sertürner tested this extract in heroic experiments on himself and his friends. However, the publication of his discovery remained unnoticed. He resumed his investigation of opium extracts after nearly 10 years, and used the new label *'morphium'* (derived from

Morpheus, the Greek god of sleep) for sleeping-inducing substance in 1817 (Tsagareli, 2018).

The endogenous opioid system is one of the most studied innate pain-relieving systems. This system consists of widely scattered neurons that produce three opioids: the beta-endorphin, met-enkephalin and leu-enkephalin, and the dynorphins. These opioids act as neurotransmitters and neuromodulators at three major classes of receptors, termed mu, delta and kappa, and produce analgesia. Like their endogenous counterparts, the opioid drugs, or opiates, act at these same receptors to produce both analgesia and undesirable side effects, and endogenous opioids are an intrinsic and essential part of the brain antinociceptive system (Azzam et al., 2019; Ballantyne, Sullivan, 2017; Dickenson, Kieffer, 2013; Holden et al., 2005; Yarnitsky, 2015).

The most straightforward part of pain processing is the transmission of injury-induced pain signals through primary afferent nociceptors arising from the dorsal root ganglion, synapsing in the dorsal horn where an immediate withdrawal reflex can be produced, and crossing to the contralateral spino-thalamic tract to the thalamus, and then to the somatosensory cortex where pain is localized and subsequent actions may be processed (Basbaum et al., 2009; Kuner, Flor, 2017).

It has recently been proposed that nociception is a fundamental physiological learning process that occurs continuously, often without concurrent pain perception. Underlying this proposal is the concept that this continuous nociception can come into consciousness due to changes in central processing, for example, in the PAG. The PAG is the main pain-relevant output pathway of the limbic system. The PAG receives projections from limbic forebrain areas, including the ACC, IC, hypothalamus, and amygdala, which respond to external stimuli and motivations. The output from the PAG alters pain transmission in the dorsal horn through the RVM. The effects may be either facilitatory or inhibitory (Ballantyne, Sullivan, 2017).

Opioids play a large role in the pain modulatory system. Opioid receptors are present in all the supraspinal pain processing sites as well as the dorsal root ganglia and dorsal horn. Activation of inhibitory GABA **supraspinal neurons by opioids accounts in large part for opioids'** analgesic effects (Lau, Vaughan, 2014b). Endogenous opioids mediate relays between the component nuclei of the pain modulatory system.

Furthermore, opioid activity triggers the dopaminergic network of the PAG and the RVM to participate in descending inhibition through dopamine D1 receptors. The concept of pain perception, as distinct from nociception, being shaped by emotional learning and perceived danger, moves us closer to understanding pain as a motivational state that consciously or unconsciously drives behaviors (Ballantyne, Sullivan, 2017).

The groundbreaking insight into ligand-receptor bind mechanism came in 1973 when Pert and Snyder identified opioid receptor sites in the brain by means of naloxone-binding studies, followed by the discovery that brain neurons synthesize opioid-like peptides that produce similar effects through actions at the same receptors (Pert, Snyder, 1973; Valentino, Volkow, 2018). Coupled with the findings that naloxone-reversible analgesia could be produced by stimulation of specific brain regions, this solidified the transformative idea that opiates act by mimicking the endogenous opioid systems. Gene cloning and brain mapping revealed three opioid peptide systems encoded by individual genes for pre-proenkephalin, pre-proopiomelanocortin and pre-prodynorphin having distinct brain distributions. Likewise, three distinct opioid receptors (OR) were cloned, mu (MOR), kappa (KOR), and delta (DOR), with different selectivities for the individual endogenous peptides and for the various opiate drugs used pharmacologically (Dickenson, Kieffer, 2013; Valentino, Volkow, 2018).

These three opioid receptors signaling systems play unique and counterbalancing roles as they relate to their regulation of pain, stress, and affect (Figure 5) (Valentino, Volkow, 2018). Though the MOR is the main target for opioid analgesics, the DOR and KOR also regulate pain and analgesia and the relative affinities of opioid analgesics for these receptors confers them unique properties. The rewarding effects of opioids also rely on the MOR, though DOR and KOR modulate them through the regulation of hedonics, mood, and stress reactivity. Specifically, while MOR agonists produce euphoria and promote stress coping, KOR agonists produce dysphoria, stress-like responses and negative affect, while agonists at DOR reduce anxiety and promote positive affect (Figure 5) (Valentino, Volkow, 2018). The multiplicity of opioid receptors inspired the design of agonists and antagonists with different potencies, efficacies and selectivities for MOR, DOR, and KOR based on structure activity relationships and with different pharmacokinetics in an effort to develop analgesics with less adverse effects. These are also being pursued as potential treatments for addiction and depression. Although promising, this strategy has yet to yield a potent opioid analgesic that is not rewarding, lacks tolerance, does not trigger physical dependence or produce respiratory depression (Darcq, Kieffer, 2018; Lutz, Kieffer, 2013; Peciña et al., 2019).

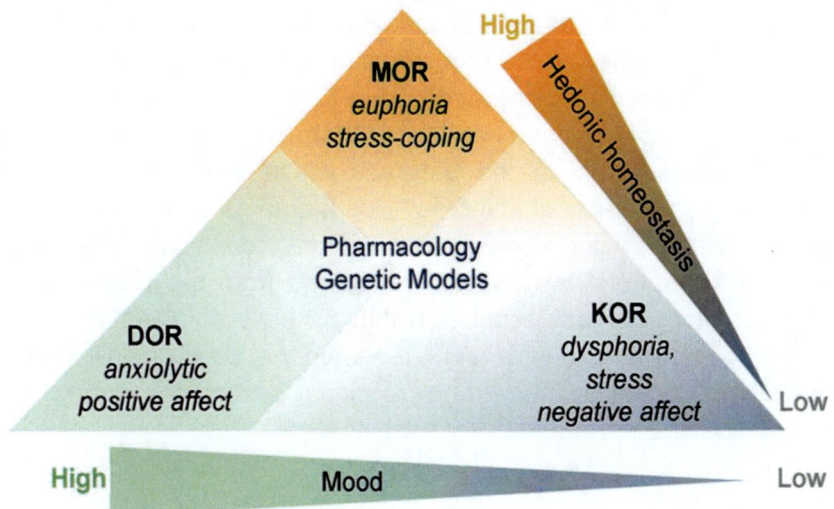

Figure 5. All MOR, KOR, and DOR are analgesics. Pharmacological studies and genetic models reveal that they are at different ends of mood and hedonic continuums. MOR agonists produce euphoria and promote stress coping. At the other end of the hedonic continuum, KOR agonists produce dysphoria and are associated with stress and negative affect. DOR is on the opposite end of the continuum describing mood and DOR agonists have anxiolytic and antidepressant activity (Reproduce from Valentino, Volkow, 2018, with permission).

The recent advances in opioid function and dysfunction and a clearer feel for the factors that can influence the efficacy of opioids form a basis for improving the clinical outcomes of opioid use. Opioids and their receptors are part of the integrated functional pharmacological repertoire of neurons in the nervous system; consequently, alteration in the status of opioid receptors and activation of other transmitter systems will interact to modulate the function of the CNS. This knowledge can be harnessed by means of combination therapy, and recognizing the potential for plasticity in opioid actions, clinical use of these drugs can be improved (Dickenson, Kieffer, 2013, Yarnitsky, 2015).

Apart from analgesia, opioid dependence and withdrawal are complex biological processes that appear to be subject to the influence of cannabinoids. The findings from basic and pre-clinical studies in rodent models highlight several potential mechanisms through which cannabinoids may modulate the phenomenon of opioid withdrawal, and call attention to the importance of cannabinoid–opioid interactions within, for example, noradrenergic brain circuits such as the coeruleo–cortical pathway. Preclinical studies that continue to explore the safest and most effective means of using cannabinoids to target disrupted noradrenergic circuits will be central to the progress within this field of research. Determining whether cannabinoids have therapeutic efficacy in clinical populations similar to that reported in animal models will be extremely important. Ultimately, the knowledge gained from the preclinical and clinical research studies described within this review highlights important and exciting new avenues for future research that continue to investigate cannabinoid effects on noradrenergic circuit dysfunction during opioid dependence and withdrawal (Scavone et al., 2013).

CANNABINOID SYSTEM

The *Cannabis sativa* plant has been used for medicinal reasons for thousands of years by different cultures. The first documentation of cannabis as a medicine appeared in China 5000 years ago when it was recommended for malaria, constipation, rheumatic pains and, mixed with wine, as a surgical analgesic. In India, more than 1000 years BC, the plant was used for various functions, such as a hypnotic and a tranquilizer useful in the treatment of anxiety, mania and hysteria. Also, the Assyrians inhaled cannabis to relieve symptoms of depression (Mechoulam, 2019).

A Greek physician Pedacius Dioscorides, between 50 and 70 AD classified different plants, including *C. sativa*, and described the benefits derived from its use in his book *De Materia Medica*. Only in the 19th century cannabis was introduced into Western medicine for its analgesic, anti-inflammatory, anti-vomiting and anti-convulsant properties (Tsagareli, 2018).

In the beginning of the 20th century, cannabis extracts were used for the treatment of mental disorders, especially as sedatives and hypnotics. After the 1930s, the medical use of cannabis significantly decreased as it was considered to be an illegal substance, its use in psychiatry was limited further. However, after the identification of the main components of cannabis and the discovery that endocannabinoid system (ECS) is able to modulate different processes in pain medicine and psychiatric disorders, the interest in the use of cannabinoids has been renewed (Hill et al., 2017; Hohmann, Rice, 2013; Jimenez, 2018; Krebs et al., 2019; Matsinu et al., 2018; Russo, Guy, 2006; Tsagareli, 2018). Finally, the medical use of cannabis extracts was approved in June 2010 by ten European countries (Kmietowicz, 2010; Di Marzo et al., 2015).

Despite its extensive history as a folk treatment for numerous health conditions, controlled clinical studies on the efficacy of cannabis have only recently begun to accumulate. The past half-century has witnessed several notable achievements in the science of cannabis, and the identification of ECS in the mammalian brain. Furthermore, interest in the utility of cannabinoids as potential analgesics has greatly increased over the past decade (Abrams, Guzman, 2015; Cristino et al., 2020; Di Marzo et al., 2015; Mun et al., 2020). In particular, neuroimaging data of pain in animal models (Da Silva, Seminowicz, 2019), and strong and consistent preclinical evidence from rodent models has suggested that cannabinoids might be a promising class of analgesics. However, efficacy data from human clinical trials in patients with noncancer pain outcomes are equivocal (Lötsch et al., 2018).

Apart from the endogenous opioid system, the second ubiquitous endogenous pain control pathway is the ECS (Figure 6) (Woodhams et al., 2017). In the past two decades, numerous tools to perturb the ECS have been developed demonstrating the potential efficacy of this approach for pain relief and for neurological disorders. However, global targeting of the ECS is also associated with undesirable results, including deleterious effects on memory, cognition, and mood, and the development of tolerance and dependence in humans (Cristino et al., 2020; Lichtman, Martin, 2005; Rubino et al., 2015; Woodhams et al., 2017). Similarly, laboratory animals exhibit both tolerance and dependence following chronic administration of cannabinoids (Lichtman, Martin, 2005).

Components of the cannabinoid system are expressed almost ubiquitously throughout nociceptive pathways, and thus targeting the system *via* exogenous cannabinoid ligands (Woodhams et al., 2017) or enhancement of endogenous communication regulating nociceptive signaling at multiple sites; in the periphery the dorsal horn of the spinal cord and in supraspinal pain-associated regions of the brain (Figure 6).

The ECS – as consisting of the cannabinoid 1 receptor (CB1) and cannabinoid 2 receptor (CB2) and of endogenous cannabinoid ligands (or endocannabinoids), and their metabolizing enzymes – is implicated in pain signaling pathways. Cannabinoids are a diverse class of biologically active constituents of cannabis or synthetic compounds, which usually have affinity for and activity at cannabinoid receptors (Soliman et al., 2019).

The first cannabinoids to be chemically characterized, delta-9-tetrahydrocannabinol (THC), and cannabidiol (CBD) were the most abundant members of this class of natural products in the dried and heated flowers of *C. sativa* varieties that are used for the production of marijuana and hemp, respectively. Accordingly, THC is responsible for the psychoactive effects of marijuana whereas CBD was found to be non-psychotropic (Di Marzo, 2018). THC acts *via* two G protein-coupled receptors (GPCRs), – CB1 and CB2 receptors, – and that CB1 is responsible for the psychoactive effects of marijuana. However, to date, no specific receptor for CBD has been identified. Several different molecular targets have been suggested to mediate distinct pharmacological effects of this cannabinoid (Di Marzo, 2018). It is interesting to note here that CBD has been traditionally used in Cannabis-based preparation; however, historically it has received far less interest as a single drug than the other components of Cannabis. Currently, CBD generates considerable interest due to its beneficial neuroprotective, antiepileptic, anxiolytic, antipsychotic, and anti-inflammatory properties. Therefore, the CBD scaffold becomes of increasing interest for medicinal chemists (Morales et al., 2017).

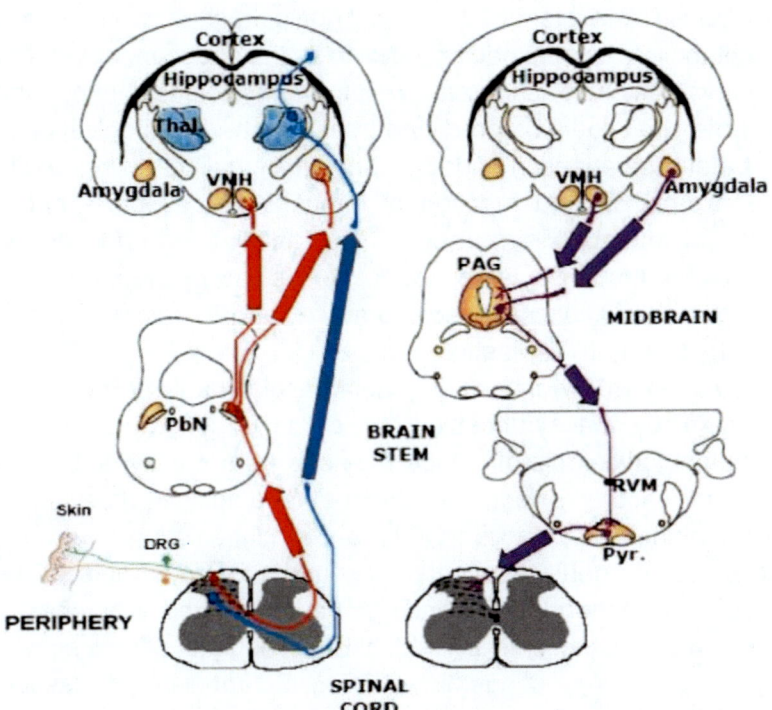

Figure 6. Schematic of ascending nociceptive pathways and sites of endogenous opioid and cannabinoid systems expression. Nociceptive stimuli are conducted from the periphery to the spinal dorsal horn (peptidergic PAF, green, and non-peptidergic PAF, yellow); then transmitted to the supraspinal regions *via* the spinothalamic tract (STT, blue) and spino-parabrachial tract (SPBT, red). The major descending modulatory control pathway (DMCP, purple) crosses the midline at the level of the medulla to spinal cord. Abbreviations: Thal., thalamus; VMH, ventromedial hypothalamus; PbN, parabrachial nucleus; PAF, primary afferent fiber; PAG, periaqueductal grey matter; RVM, rostral ventro-medial medulla; Pyr., pyramidal tract; DRG, dorsal root ganglion (Adapted from Woodhams et al., 2017, with permission).

The identification of CB1, predominantly expressed in the brain and CB2, expressed mainly in immune cells and during inflammatory injury in the CNS, led to the isolation and characterization of endogenous ligands for these proteins. The first *N*-arachidonoyl-ethanolamine (AEA) was named '*anandamide*' for the Sanskrit word for 'bliss.' The second is 2-arachidonoylglycerol (2-AG), both of which were named the endocannabinoids (ECs), and of five main enzymes for their biosynthesis and inactivation. This system of two signaling lipids, their two receptors and their metabolic enzymes became known as the endocannabinoid system (ECS) and was soon assigned a wealth of physiological roles that went far beyond what could be predicted from the pharmacological actions of THC. Later, alterations in endocannabinoid signaling, owing to changes in the expression and function of cannabinoid receptors and endocannabinoid metabolic enzymes, as well as modified endocannabinoid tissue concentrations, were found to be associated with diverse pathological conditions (Console-Bram et al., 2012; Di Marzo, 2018; Mallipeddi et al., 2017; Mastinu et al., 2018).

In addition, ECs work as key regulators of synaptic transmission and plasticity. They are synthesized "on demand" following physiological and/or pathological stimuli. Once released from postsynaptic neurons, ECs typically act as retrograde messengers to activate presynaptic type 1st cannabinoid receptors (CB1) and induce short- or long-term depression of neurotransmitter release. Besides this canonical mechanism of action, recent findings have revealed a number of less conventional mechanisms by which ECs regulate neural activity and synaptic function, suggesting that EC-mediated plasticity is mechanistically more diverse than anticipated. These mechanisms include non-retrograde signaling, signaling *via* astrocytes, and participation in long-term potentiation in some brain areas such as hippocampus, striatum, and neocortex. Thus, EC signaling may lead to different forms of synaptic plasticity through activation of a plethora of mechanisms, which provide further complexity to the functional consequences of EC signalment (Araque et al., 2017).

Since the discovery of the cannabinoid receptors and their endogenous ligands, the ECS has been regularly regarded as a putative target for the treatment of several pathologies, including neurodegenerative diseases (Alzheimer's disease, Parkinson's disease, Huntington's disease, etc.), cancer, neuropathic and inflammatory pain, obesity, etc. Nevertheless, the potential clinical uses of cannabinoids remain strongly limited by the unacceptable adverse effects of cannabis including its psychotropic action (Abrams, Goozman, 2015; Krebs et al., 2019) or tolerance, dependence, and withdrawal symptoms upon drug cessation (Lichtman, Martin, 2005).

While remarkable advances in the development of highly selective agonists have emerged during this last decade, present studies indicate that specificity in cannabinoid-mediated functions is not only achieved by the pharmacological profile of the ligand used but also depends on cell/model-related parameters. Therefore, the ability to selectively manipulate different physiological functions by targeting either a subpopulation of receptors or a defined associated signaling cascade will certainly constitute the basis of novel and promising therapeutic approaches. Along this line, the observation that some THC derivatives are equally potent to THC in inducing anti-nociception, while being 30–40 fold less potent in inducing hypothermia, hypoactivity or catalepsy is encouraging. Certainly, a more thorough characterization of the versatile nature of cannabinoid signaling is essential to optimize the development of cannabinoid ligands as therapeutically safe drugs (Bosier et al., 2010; Mallipeddi et al., 2017; Mastinu et al., 2018).

Whereas waiting for effective and safe non-brain-penetrant analogs, CB1 antagonists could be repositioned for use in patients with a low risk of developing depression relative to individuals who are obese [the population in which rimonabant (zimulti, an anorectic anti-obesity drug) was unsafe] or for orphan and otherwise untreatable diseases. Exploiting the positive and negative allosteric sites in CB1 and CB2 could be useful in diseases such as chronic pain, cancer, anxiety, depression and schizophrenia and in metabolic and neuro-inflammatory disorders. In this respect, recently identified endogenous negative allosteric modulators of cannabinoid receptors, like some hemopressin (an inverse agonist at CB1 receptors) analogs and pregnenolone, could provide starting points for new treatments for addiction disorders and cannabis and synthetic cannabinoid intoxication. Finally, the thorough biomolecular investigation of gut microbiome – endocannabinoidome interactions will likely lead to new drugs, which could include synthetic analogs of multi-target endocannabinoid-like mediators designed to have drug-like properties (Di Marzo, 2018).

OPIOID AND CANNABINOID SYSTEMS INTERACTION

As stated above, among several pharmacological properties, analgesia is the most common feature shared by either opioid or cannabinoid systems. Cannabinoids and opioids are distinct drug classes that have been historically used separately or in combination to treat different pain states. Indeed, it is widely known that activation of either opioid or cannabinoid systems produce antinociceptive properties in different pain models. Moreover, several biochemical, molecular and pharmacological studies support the existence of reciprocal interactions between both systems, suggesting a common underlying mechanism. Further studies have demonstrated that the endogenous opioid system could be involved in cannabinoid antinociception and recent data have also provided evidence for a role of the ECS in opioid antinociception. These interactions may lead to additive or even synergistic antinociceptive effects, emphasizing their clinical relevance in humans in order to enhance analgesic effects with lower doses and consequently fewer undesirable side effects (Abrams et al., 2011; Desroches, Beaulieu, 2010).

In the next work of Desroches and coauthors (2014) studied involvement of the cannabinoid system in morphine induced analgesia. In both phases of the formalin test, intra paw and intrathecal morphine produced similar antinociceptive effects in C57BL/6, cannabinoid type 1 and type 2 receptor wild-type (respectively *cnr1*WT and *cnr2*WT) mice. In *cnr1* and *cnr2* knockout (KO) mice, at the dose used the antinociceptive effect of intra paw morphine in the inflammatory phase of the formalin test was decreased by 87% and 76%, respectively. Similarly, the antinociceptive effect of 0.1 μg spinal morphine in the inflammatory phase was abolished in *cnr1*KO mice and decreased by 90% in *cnr2*KO mice. Interestingly, the antinociceptive effect of morphine in the acute phase of the formalin test was only reduced in *cnr1*KO mice. Notably, systemic morphine administration produced similar analgesia in all genotypes, in both the formalin and the hot water immersion tail-flick tests. Because the pattern of expression of the mu opioid receptor (MOR), its binding properties and its G protein coupling remained unchanged across genotypes, it is unlikely that the loss of morphine analgesia in the *cnr1*KO and *cnr2*KO mice is the consequence of MOR malfunction or down-regulation due to the absence of its heterodimerization with either the CB1 or the CB2 receptors, at least at the level of the spinal cord (Desroches et al., 2014).

In this regard, it is suggested that THC enhances some antinociceptive effects of MOR agonists, suggesting that cannabinoids might be combined with opioids to treat pain without increasing, and possibly decreasing, abuse. The degree to which cannabinoids enhance antinociceptive effects of opioids varies across drugs insofar as THC and the synthetic cannabinoid receptor agonist CP55940 increase the potency of some MOR agonists (e.g., fentanyl) more than others (e.g., nalbuphine). It is not known whether interactions between cannabinoids and opioids vary similarly for other (abuse-related) effects. It was examined whether THC and CP55940 differentially impact the discriminative stimulus effects of fentanyl and nalbuphine in monkeys (n=4) discriminating 0.01 mg/kg of fentanyl subcutaneously (s.c.) from saline. Fentanyl (0.00178–0.0178 mg/kg) and nalbuphine (0.01–0.32 mg/kg) dose-dependently increased drug-lever responding. Neither THC (0.032–1.0 mg/kg) nor CP55940 (0.0032–0.032 mg/kg) enhanced the discriminative stimulus effects of fentanyl or nalbuphine; however, doses of THC and CP55940 that shifted then nalbuphine dose-effect curve markedly to the right and/or down were less effective or ineffective in shifting the fentanyl dose-effect curve. The MOR antagonist naltrexone (0.032 mg/kg) attenuated the discriminative stimulus effects of fentanyl and nalbuphine similarly (Maguire, France, 2016). These data indicate that the discriminative stimulus effects of nalbuphine are more sensitive to attenuation by cannabinoids than those of fentanyl. That the discriminative stimulus effects of some opioids are more susceptible to modification by drugs from other classes has implications for developing maximally effective therapeutic drug mixtures with reduced abuse liability.

Presently, it is well known that opioid and cannabinoid receptors are major targets for many drugs of abuse and widely-used analgesics. These receptor systems are known to mediate common signaling pathways central to clinical issues of tolerance, dependence and addiction. Drugs that target both the CB1 and MOR systems possess shared pharmacological profiles. Agonists of both receptor types have been shown to cause antinociception, sedation, hypotension, motor depression, and drug reward/reinforcement (Scavone et al., 2013). Cannabinoids may be able to modulate opioid function at a number of different levels within the cell, ranging from direct receptor associations, to alterations in endogenous peptide release, or to post-receptor interactions *via* shared signal transduction pathways. Evidence of these interactions can be observed through the various studies demonstrating cross-tolerance, mutual/synergistic potentiation, and receptor cross-talk. Importantly, drugs that target the cannabinoid system often seem to affect the opioid system in tandem (Kazantzis et al., 2016).

A very interesting investigation was carried out on cannabinoid – opioid interaction in chronic pain. Twenty-one patients with chronic pain, on a regimen of twice-daily doses of sustained release morphine or oxycodone were enrolled in the study and admitted for a 5-day inpatient stay. Participants were asked to inhale vaporized cannabis for 5 days. Blood sampling was performed at 12-h intervals on days 1 and 5. The extent of chronic pain was also assessed daily. Pharmacokinetic investigations revealed no significant change in the area under the plasma concentration – time curves for either morphine or oxycodone after exposure to cannabis. Pain was significantly decreased after the addition of vaporized cannabis. The authors therefore concluded that vaporized cannabis augmented the analgesic effects of opioids without significantly altering plasma opioid levels, and this combination of analgesics, thus, may allow for opioid treatment at lower doses with fewer side effects (Abrams et al., 2011).

In the other investigation, the opioid agonist morphine reduced the sciatic nerve chronic constriction injury (CCI)-induced mechanical and cold allodynia and produced motor incoordination, in a dose dependent manner. The pan-cannabinoid receptor agonist WIN55212 also reduced CCI-induced allodynia and produced motor incoordination, catalepsy and sedation, in a dose-dependent manner. It was interesting that when administered together, WIN55212 and morphine reduced allodynia in a synergistic manner but had only an additive effect on motor incoordination. These findings indicated that administration of a combination of a non-selective opioid and cannabinoid receptor agonist synergistically reduced nerve injury-induced allodynia, while producing side effects in an additive manner. This suggests that this combination treatment has an improved anti-allodynic potency and therapeutic index in a neuropathic pain model (Kazantzis et al., 2016).

However, more clinical studies are needed for the dedication, credibility, and expertise to carry out the work required addressing the issues of combination use of opioids and cannabinoids. Replication and confirmation of such small studies, dose-finding studies, abuse liability studies, and studies of the effects on cognition and driving, using standardized cannabis materials in well-defined clinical populations, are desperately needed to respond to the concerns and claims on both sides of the medical marijuana debate. In these regards, most of the safety data for cannabis use to date come from large-scale epidemiological or small interventional studies in volunteers, and it is tempting but erroneous to extrapolate these results to the clinical population without considering differences in dose, underlying comorbidities, concomitant medications, and attempts to alleviate target symptoms that separate the true medical cannabis user from the casual recreational cannabis user (Ware, 2011).

Recently preclinical studies have provided robust evidence of the opioid-sparing effect of cannabinoids. It means that cannabinoids, when co-administered with opioids, may enable reduced opioid doses without loss of analgesic efficacy (i.e., an opioid-sparing effect). In particular, preclinical studies support the opioid-sparing effect of THC. Thus, opioid-sparing medications may have enormous clinical relevance by enabling effective pain treatment with lower opioid doses and a potential reduction in opioid-related mortality (Nielsen et al., 2017). However, the potential benefits of cannabis-based medicine (herbal cannabis, plant-derived or synthetic THC, THC/CBD oro-mucosal spray), THC, CBD in chronic neuropathic pain might be outweighed by their potential harms. However, the quality of evidence for pain relief outcomes reflects the exclusion of participants with a history of substance abuse and other significant comorbidities from the studies, together with their small sample sizes (Mücke et al., 2018).

Chapter 4

NON-OPIOID TOLERANCE

The relatively high efficacy of opioids, which have associated risks of addiction, tolerance, and dependence, for the management of acute, chronic and terminal pain has been a major driver of the present opioid crisis, together with the availability, over-prescription, and diversion of these drugs. To deal successfully with this opioid crisis, pharmacy needs to discover novel analgesics whose mechanisms do not involve the MOR but that have high analgesic potency and low risk of adverse effects, particularly no abuse liability and tolerance (Bannister et al., 2017). There are only a rather limited number of targets on which drugs act to produce clinically meaningful analgesia (Table 1). In most cases, the molecular target of these analgesics was only elucidated well after the discovery of the analgesic action of the compound, as for morphine or salicylate drugs, and in many cases the analgesic action was found secondary to some other clinical indication (anti-inflammatory, antiepileptic, anesthetic or antidepressant (Woolf, 2020).

Ideally, it is necessary to match the treatment with conditions in which particular targets are prominent and detectable drivers in the patient pain experiences. Part of the diagnostic effort, therefore, needs to be elucidating what mechanisms are causing the pain in an individual patient and using this information to identify targets for therapeutic intervention. A simple illustration of this is COX-2, which is induced in macrophages early in inflammation and contributes to peripheral sensitization. Interestingly, COX-2 is also induced in neurons in the spinal cord, where it contributes to central sensitization. In the absence of the peripheral and central induction, the target is not available, and NSAIDs will have no on-target effect (Woolf, 2020).

Table 1. Analgesic targets providing clinically validated efficacy

Targets	Analgesics (Drug Function)
Alpha2-delta1 calcium channel	Gabapentin (antiepileptic)
Cav2.2 calcium channel	Ziconotide
CGRP	Erenumab (migraine)
COX-2	NSAIDs/COX-2 inhibitors (anti-inflammatory)
Mu-opioid receptor	Morphine/opioids
NMDA receptor	Ketamine (dissociative anesthetic)
Sepiapterin reductase	Sulfasalazine (anti-inflammatory)
Serotonin-norepinephrine reuptake	Duloxetine (antidepressant)
Voltage-gated sodium channel	Carbamazepine (antiepileptic)
5-HT1B/D serotonin receptor agonists	Triptans (migraine)

Abbreviations: Cav2.2, voltage-gated calcium channel 2.2; CGRP, calcitonin gene-related peptide; COX-2, cyclooxygenase-2; 5-HT, 5-hydroxytryptamine (serotonin); NMDA, N-methyl-D-aspartate receptor; NSAID, non-steroidal anti-inflammatory drug (adapted from Woolf, 2020).

TOLERANCE TO NON-STEROIDAL ANTI-INFLAMMATORY DRUGS

Nowadays, non-opioid analgesics are widely used for pain relief in general, in palliative medicine as well in particular. However, there is a lack of evidence-based recommendations addressing the efficacy, tolerability, and safety of non-opioids in this field (Schüchen et al., 2018; Tsagareli, Tsiklauri, 2012; Tsiklauri et al., 2016).

Almost similar, non-opioid treatments for chronic breathlessness are less studied than morphine and morphine-related medications, although evidence is emerging in relation to some options. Currently, there is insufficient evidence to recommend non-opioids in the routine treatment of chronic breathlessness. There is a need to find agents, new as well as re-purposed, that can be used as alternative therapies to opioids for chronic breathlessness for people who are unable to tolerate morphine (Barbetta et al., 2017).

The NSAIDs, COX-2 inhibitors (coxibs) and other non-opioid analgesics are important in management, both on and off prescription. They are classified into three groups according to their physio-chemical properties, their selectivity for two COX-1 and COX-2 isoforms, and their clinical actions. NSAIDs are acidic compounds that inhibit the two COXs with similar high potency and efficacy. In addition to their analgesic and antipyretic effect, they exert profound anti-inflammatory actions. The second group comprises selective inhibitors of COX-2. Because COX-2 produces most of the prostaglandins that contribute to inflammation, nociceptive sensitization and fever, coxibs are antipyretic, analgesic, and anti-inflammatory. The third group comprises classic non-acidic antipyretic analgesics – such as dipyrone/metamizole and acetaminophen/paracetamol which are relatively weak inhibitors of COXs *in vitro* (Moore, McQuay, 2013; Zeilhofer, Brune, 2013).

On the other hand, combination therapy of opioids and non-opioids is a well-established clinical pharmaco-therapeutic strategy for the treatment of various pain states. The combination of MOR agonists with non-MOR agonists may increase the analgesic potency of MOR agonists, reduce the development of tolerance and dependence, reduce the diversion and abuse, overdose, and reduce other clinically significant side effects associated with prolonged opioid use such as constipation. Overall, the combination therapy approach could substantially improve the therapeutic profile of MOR agonists (Li, 2019).

As stated above, NSAIDs are the most widely used analgesics mostly in the treatment of not severe pain. These drugs have analgesic, antipyretic, and at higher doses, anti-inflammatory actions. Aspirin (acetylsalicylic acid) as the first NSAID was produced in 1853 by German-French chemist Charles Frédéric Gerhardt but then has been largely replaced by drugs that are less toxic to gastro-intestinal tract, e.g. paracetamol, ibuprofen, ketorolac, naproxen, lornoxicam. NSAIDs produce their effects by inhibiting cyclooxygenases (mostly COX-1), key enzymes in the production of prostaglandins. The latter are one of the mediators released at sites of inflammation. They do not themselves cause pain but they potentiated the pain caused by other mediators, e.g. histamine, serotonin, bradykinin (Tsagareli, Tsiklauri, 2012).

The analgesic effects of non-opioid pain-relieving drugs are due to their action on the brainstem structures and peripheral tissues. Their action on the latter has been far better studied than on the CNS. It is known that non-opioid analgesics cause antinociception through the three main parts of human body, in particular, on the level of inflammation carrying peripheral tissues, spinal cord and brainstem. It is supposed that on the brainstem level the non-opioids accomplish their pain-relieving action through activation of the PAG. The latter has been considered as the descending, down-stream pain control system, which blocks the pain signals on the level of spinal cord dorsal horn neurons (Fields et al., 2014; Heinricher, Fields, 2013; Heinricher, Ingram, 2009; Keay, Bandler, 2009; Ossipov et al., 2014; Ren, Dubner, 2009; Tsagareli, Tsiklauri, 2012).

On the one hand, NSAIDs cause inhibition of the pain sensitive, nociceptive neurons and reduction of nociceptive responses *via* action on the spinal cord, in unanesthetized animals and in tumor carrying patients (Bannister et al., 2017; Moore, McQuay, 2013; Schüchen et al., 2018; Salas et al., 2016, 2018). On the other hand, as shown by our and Vanegas laboratory findings, the NSAIDs, such as ketorolac, dipyrone or analgin (metamizole), lysine-acetylsalicylate (LASA) and xefocam, under conditions of systemic administration, activate the pain downstream control system and inhibit the spinal nociceptive reflexes (Pernia-Andrade, et al, 2004; Tortorici et al., 2009; Tsagareli, Tsiklauri, 2012; Tsiklauri, Tsagareli, 2006; Tsiklauri et al., 2009, 2011). Interestingly, the downstream nociceptive inhibition induced by intraperitoneal (i.p.) injection of metamizole, ketorolac and lornoxicam is mediated by involvement of endogenous opioidergic circuitry, since the latter is blocked by systemic administration of naloxone (opioid receptor antagonist) (Hernandez-Delgadillo, Cruz, 2006; Tsiklauri, Tsagareli, 2006; Tsiklauri et al., 2009; 2011; 2016).

Our and other colleagues' studies for last two decades demonstrated that NSAIDs, in the case of their repeated and prolonged use, elicit the opioid-like effect, tolerance. In particular, repeated injections of metamizole, ketorolac and xefocam lead to a gradual attenuation of antinociceptive efficacy that is evidenced by tolerance toward them and cross-tolerance to i.p. morphine injections (Tsagareli, Tsiklauri, 2012; Tsiklauri, Tsagareli, 2006; Tsiklauri et al, 2009; Vanegas, Tortorici, 2002). Moreover, systemic naloxone completely prevented the analgesic effects of these non-opioid drugs in juvenile and adult rats. In addition, in morphine tolerant juvenile and adult rats we revealed effects of cross-tolerance to analgin (metamizole), ketorolac and lornoxicam (Tsiklauri et al., 2009). Finally, during systemic administration of naloxone the drug withdrawal syndrome is in evidence (Tortorici, Vanegas, 2000).

We have recently shown in acute pain models of rats using the tail flick (TF) and hot plate (HP) tests, microinjections of NSAIDs, analgin, diclofenac, ketorolac, and lornoxicam in the PAG, the central nucleus of amygdala (CeA), and the nucleus raphe magnus (NRM), induces antinociception and the effects of tolerance and cross-tolerance to morphine in repeated microinjections (Gurtskaia et al, 2014a; Tsagareli et al, 2009; 2010, 2011; Tsiklauri et al, 2010; 2011; 2016). These findings strongly support the suggestion of endogenous opioids involvement in NSAIDs antinociception and tolerance in the descending pain-control system (Tortorici et al, 2009; Tortorici, Vanegas, 2000; Vanegas et al, 2010; Tsagareli, Tsiklauri, 2012; Tsiklauri et al., 2016).

Furthermore, we have recently revealed that microinjection of diclofenac, ketorolac, and lornoxicam into the dorsal hippocampus (DH) leads to the development of antinociceptive tolerance in rats. We found that microinjection of these NSAIDs into the DH induces antinociception as revealed by a latency increase in the TF and HP tests compared to controls treated with saline into the DH. Subsequent tests on consecutive three days, however, showed that the antinociceptive effect of NSAIDs progressively decreased, suggesting tolerance developed to this effect of NSAIDs. Both pre- and post-treatments with the opioid antagonist naloxone into the DH significantly reduced the antinociceptive effect of NSAIDs in both acute pain tests. Our data indicate that microinjection of NSAIDs into the DH induces antinociception which is mediated *via* the endogenous opioid system and exhibits tolerance (Gurtskaia et al, 2014a; Tsiklauri et al., 2016).

Finally, we have just recently reported the development of tolerance to the analgesic effects of NSAIDs diclofenac, ketorolac and lornoxicam in one of chronic inflammatory pain models such as the formalin test (FT). Rats were tested for antinociception following i.p. injection of

NSAIDs in thermal paw withdrawal (Hargreaves) test and mechanical paw withdrawal (von Frey) test. Our data have shown that after i.p. injection of each drug, the thermal paw withdrawal latency and mechanical paw withdrawal threshold were significantly elevated on the first day followed by a progressive decrease of these indices over the 4-day period, i.e., tolerance was developed. It is noteworthy that the NSAID tolerant groups of rats exhibited a strong hyperalgesia unlike non-tolerant groups. Pretreatment with naloxone (i.p.) completely prevented the analgesic effects of these three NSAIDs in two behavioral assays. These findings support the notion that analgesic and tolerance effects of NSAIDs are mediated *via* endogenous opioid system along the descending pain control mechanism (Tsiklauri et al., 2017). Interestingly, it has been previously shown that inflammation of the rat's paw (an intraplantar injection of carrageenan) was attenuated by intra-PAG microinjection of dipyrone (metamizole) and this antinociceptive effect of dipyrone was reduced by a microinjection of AM-251, an antagonist at the CB1 cannabinoid receptor, either into PAG or RVM (Escobar et al., 2012).

The given findings in quite a new light pose the question about the development of NSAIDs-induced tolerance, since the latter phenomenon is elicited by opioids, i.e., morphine and other opioid drugs. Obviously, NSAIDs induced tolerance, is likely to be related with endogenous pain relieving (antinociceptive) opioid and cannabinoid systems. Thus, the study of the mechanisms of NSAIDs action is extremely topical and has significant implications for medical practice in as much development of tolerance to non-opioids alongside with the drug withdrawal syndrome that may entail serious medical and social complications.

Chapter 5

ANTINOCICEPTIVE TOLERANCE TO NSAIDS IN ANTERIOR CINGULATE CORTEX

The brain, which harbors numerous cortical and subcortical structures that are activated *via* three major ascending pathways, spino-reticular, spino-mesencephalic and spino-thalamic upon peripheral nociceptive stimulation, is crucial for pain perception. A brain network analysis suggested that there are broad-ranging structures responsible to pain emotions with a focus on insular and cingulate cortices, hypothalamus, and hippocampus (Kuner, Flor, 2017). Studies of the emotional and motivational basis of pain reveal a diverse and complex set of processes by which the affective experience of pain is realized. In particular, the perception of both pain intensity and aversiveness is the complex process by which the brain constructs the sensory and emotional sensation of pain and challenges any standard "perception-action" model (Seymour, Dolan, 2013).

The first anatomical, physiological and behavioral investigations have demonstrated the important role of the brain limbic system in the affective-motivational component of pain. Some animal studies and clinical evidence have shown the importance of the ACC in affective aspects of pain (Craig, 2006). It is well known that the ACC is involved in pain perception primarily receiving extensive projections from the medio-dorsal thalamic nucleus and broadly connects with relevant regions of the descending pain modulation system (Xiao, Zhang, 2018). A projection from the spinal dorsal horn through the medial/intra-laminar thalamic nuclei to the ACC has been proposed to process information on pain-related unpleasantness. In addition to contributing to the immediate affective consequences of noxious stimulation, the "ACC system" may contribute to the avoidance learning that sometimes follows as a secondary reaction to pain (Johansen et al., 2001). However, the mechanisms of the ACC involvement in pain have yet to be elaborated (Xiao, Zhang, 2018).

In this study provided here we hypothesized that the analgesic effects of the three NSAIDs, diclofenac, ketorolac, and lornoxicam (xefocam) microinjected into the rostral ACC (rACC) would exhibit tolerance mediated *via* endogenous opioids (see methodologies in detail, the chapter 8).

TOLERANCE TO ANTINOCICEPTIVE EFFECTS OF NSAIDS IN ACC

The microinjection sites of inserted cannulas were histologically verified and plotted according to Paxinos and Watson (1997) stereotaxic atlas coordinates. Representative microinjection sites are shown in Figure 7. In the first set of experiments we found that microinjection of NSAIDs into the rACC produced antinociception as detected by a latency increase in TF and HP compared to the baseline control of intact rats and a control group with saline microinjected into the same site as well. The repeated measure analysis of variance (rMANOVA) revealed that the TF latency significantly increased for diclofenac [$F(9, 20) = 24.222$, $P < 0.0001$], ketorolac [$F(9, 20) = 71.399$, $P < 0.0001$], and lornoxicam [$F(9, 20) = 101.13$, $P < 0.0001$], respectively, but not for the saline group [$F(9, 20) = 0.4148$, $P = 0.7955$, not significant]. The TF latency differences between NSAIDs-treated groups and the saline group by Dunnett's test were significant in the first experimental day for diclofenac ($t = 3.608$, $P < 0.01$), ketorolac ($t = 3.424$, $P < 0.01$), and xefocam ($t = 3.741$, $P < 0.01$), respectively (Figure 8A). We found similar significant differences in the HP latencies for diclofenac [$F(9, 20) = 29.045$, $P < 0.0001$], for ketorolac [$F(9,20) = 55.307$, $P < 0.0001$], and for lornoxicam [$F(9,20) = 90.93$, $P < 0.0001$], respectively, but not for saline control [$F(9,20) = 1.299$, $P = 0.3123$, not significant]. The HP latency differences between NSAIDs treated groups and the control group by Dunnett's test were significant in the first experimental day for diclofenac (t = 2.687, P < 0.05) and lornoxicam (t = 2.728, P < 0.05), but not for ketorolac (t = 1.846, P > 0.05) (Figure 8B).

Subsequent NSAIDs microinjections caused progressively less antinociception, so by day 4 there was no effect, similar to saline microinjections for both the TF and the HP tests, i.e. induced tolerance. By the second experimental day the TF latency differences between NSAIDs treated groups and the saline group were significant only for lornoxicam (t = 3.066, P < 0.05) (Figure 8A). There were not significant differences between NSAIDs treated groups and the control in the HP test for the second experimental day (Figure 8B).

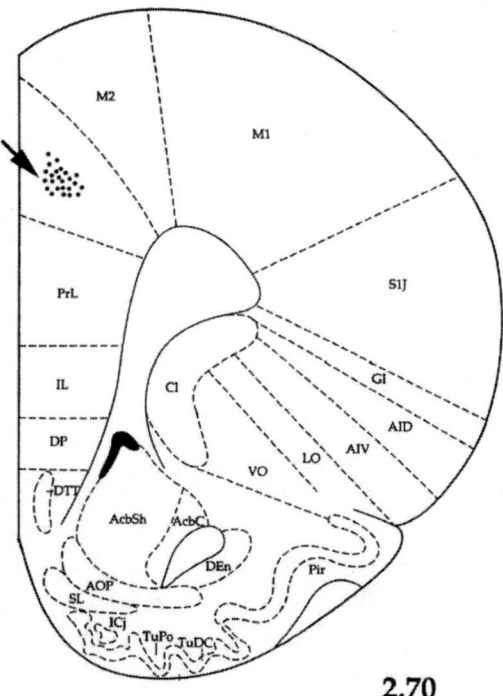

Figure 7. A serial coronal section of the rat brain showing placement microinjections unilaterally in the ACC (the black arrow) by Paxinos and Watson (1997) atlas coordinates.

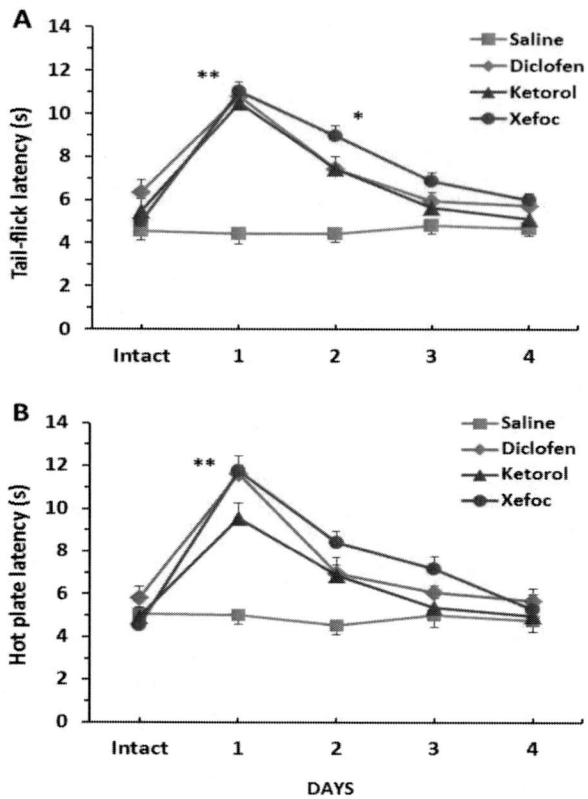

Figure 8. Microinjections of NSAIDs into the ACC for 4 consecutive days result in a progressive decrease in TF (A) and HP (B) latencies as compared to control. * - $P < 0.05$, ** - $P < 0.01$.

In the second set of experiments, we tested if pretreatment with a non-selective opioid receptor antagonist naloxone prevents antinociception induced by NSAIDs microinjected into the ACC. Pretreatment with naloxone completely prevented the analgesic effects of diclofenac, ketorolac, and lornoxicam (xefocam) in the TF test (Figure 9). The differences between NSAIDs injected and naloxone injected groups are not significant [ANOVA: $F(3,32) = 1.419$, $P = 0.2552$, not significant] The same results are in the HP test for diclofenac, ketorolac, and xefocam, respectively (Figure 10) [ANOVA: $F(3,32) = 1.829$, $P = 0.1618$, not significant].

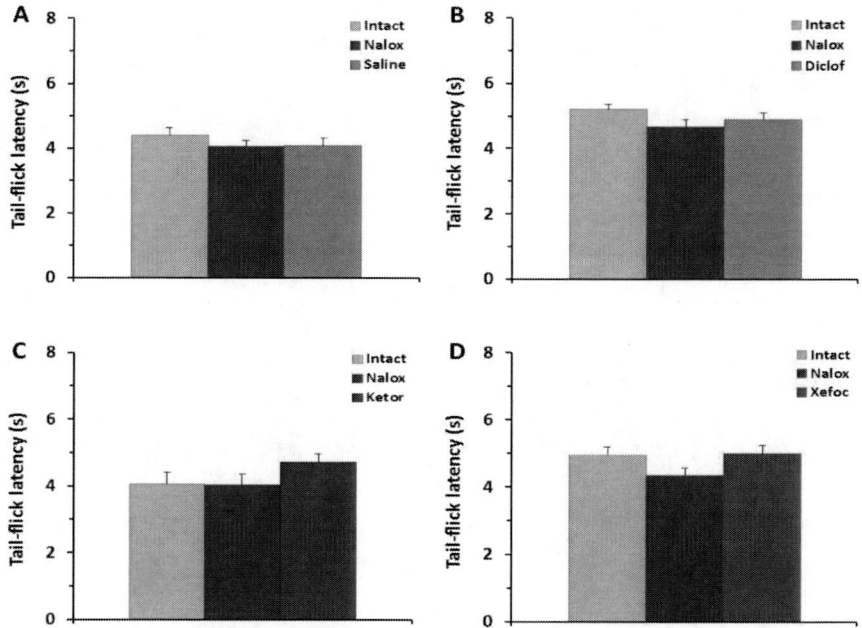

Figure 9. Pretreatment with naloxone before microinjections of NSAIDs into the rACC results in prevention of NSAID-induced antinociception in TF latency for diclofenac (B), ketorolac (C), and xefocam (D), respectively. Control experiments of pretreatment with naloxone before microinjection of saline into the rACC do not significantly change TF latency (A).

Special control testing with naloxone microinjections into the ACC followed by saline statistically did not change the latency to respond in the TF [ANOVA: $F(2,15) = 1.301$, $P = 0.3012$, not significant] (Figure 9A), and HP [ANOVA: $F(2,15) = 0.2939$, $P = 0.2939$, not significant] tests, respectively (Figure 10A).

The data reported in this study demonstrate that microinjection of commonly used NSAIDs, diclofenac, ketorolac and lornoxicam into the rostral part of ACC induces antinociception. These findings are in resemblance with the results of our and other colleagues' previous investigations in an acute pain model with TF and HP tests, and in which metamizole, lornoxicam, ketorolac or lysine-acetylsalicylate were given systemically or microinjected into the PAG (Pernia-Andrade et al., 2004; Tortorici et al., 2009; Vanegas, Tortorici, 2007; Tsiklauri et al., 2010; Tortorici, Vanegas, 2000), into the CeA (Tsagareli, Tsiklauri, 2012;

Tsagareli et al., 2010), and the NRM (Tsagareli, Tsiklauri, 2012; Tsagareli et al., 2011; Tsiklauri et al., 2016). In the other investigation, responses of spinal dorsal horn wide-dynamic range neurons of rats to mechanical noxious stimulation of a hindpaw were strongly inhibited by intravenous metamizole (Telleria-Diaz, 2010).

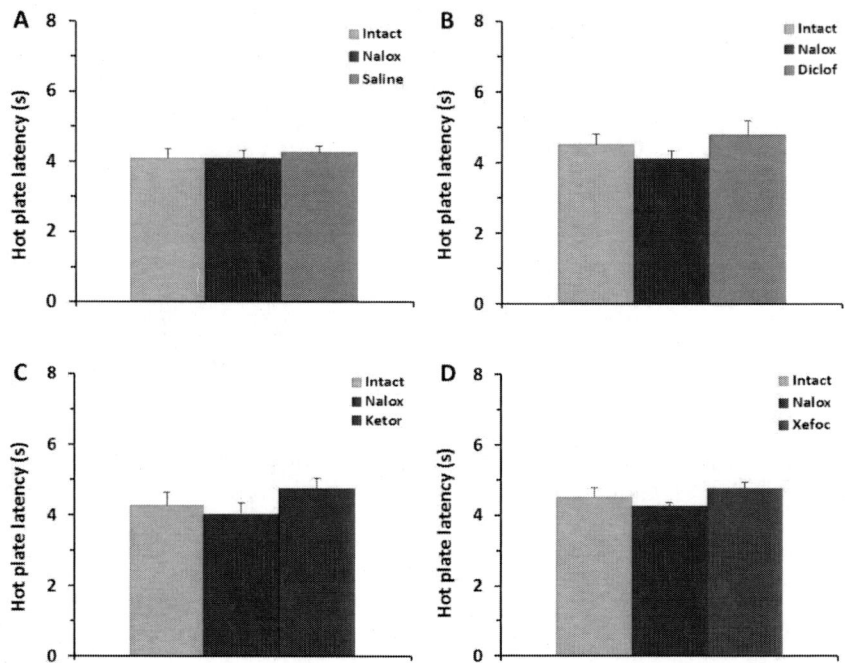

Figure 10. Pretreatment with naloxone before microinjections of NSAIDs into the rACC results in prevention of NSAID-induced antinociception in HP latency for diclofenac (B), ketorolac (C), and xefocam (D), respectively. Control experiments of pretreatment with naloxone before microinjection of saline into the rACC do not significantly change HP latency (A).

More importantly, repeated administrations of these NSAIDs into the rACC over a period of 4 days resulted in a progressive decrease in antinociceptive effectiveness, i.e., development of tolerance, reminiscent of that induced by opiates (Pernia-Andrade et al., 2004; Tortorici et al., 2003; 2004; Tsagareli, Tsiklauri, 2012; Tsiklauri et al., 2010). The present data confirm our previous results in which development of tolerance was observed to the analgesic effects of diclofenac, ketorolac and lornoxicam (xefocam) microinjected into the DH of rats. After injection of each drug, a progressive decrease in TF and HP latency (i.e., tolerance) was noticed over the 4-day period (Gurtskaia et al., 2014a; Tsiklauri et al., 2016).

The mechanism producing tolerance to NSAIDs can be due to the participation of endogenous opioids (Dickenson, Kieffer, 2013; Henricher, Fields, 2013; Tsagareli, Tsiklauri, 2012; Vanegas et al., 2010). Here we clearly showed that pretreatment of a non-selective opioid receptor antagonist naloxone significantly diminishes NSAIDs-induced antinociception. These findings confirm our previous evidence where pretreatment with naloxone prevented antinociceptive effects of metamizole, ketorolac and lornoxicam in juvenile and adult rats. Moreover, in morphine-tolerant juvenile and adult rats we revealed effects of cross-tolerance to metamizole, ketorolac and xefocam (Tsiklauri et al., 2010). As stated above, NSAIDs antinociception in the DH was reduced by pre- and post-treatment with naloxone (Gurtskaia et al., 2014a; Tsiklauri et al., 2016). Just recently we showed that systemic (i.p.) pretreatment with naloxone completely prevented the analgesic effects of NSAIDs (diclofenac, ketorolac and lornoxicam, i.p.) in thermal paw withdrawal (Hargreaves) test and mechanical paw withdrawal (von Frey) test in an inflammatory pain model, the formalin test (Tsiklauri et al., 2017). These and the present data also confirm previous results that anti-nociception induced by systemic metamizole involves endogenous opioids that can be blocked by naloxone at the levels of the PAG, NRM and spinal dorsal horn (Vazquez, 2005), as well as other findings that endogenous opioids are involved in the potentiation of analgesia observed with a combination of morphine plus dipyrone (Hernández-Delgadillo, Cruz, 2006). These data suggest a role for endogenous opioidergic descending pain control circuits. The latter consists of the brainstem pain modulatory network with critical links in the PAG and RVM (Heinricher, Fields, 2013; Heinricher, Ingram, 2009; Vanegas et al., 2010; Vazques et al., 2007).

In conclusions, here we have demonstrated that administration of diclofenac, ketorolac and lornoxicam, widely used non-opioid, NSAID analgesics, into the rostral part of the ACC, induces antinociception in rats. When administered repeatedly, tolerance developed to the antinociceptive effects of these drugs. The present findings support the concept that the development of tolerance to the antinociceptive effects of NSAIDs is mediated *via* an endogenous opioid system possibly involving descending pain modulatory systems.

ENDOGENOUS OPIOID SYSTEM IS INVOLVED IN NSAIDS – INDUCED ANTINOCICEPTION

As stated above, it is well established that the endogenous opioid system is involved in the pathophysiology of pain and plays a key role in pain control. In this work we investigated the central brain mechanisms of four NSAIDs (diclofenac, ketorolac, ketoprofen, and lornoxicam) antinociception in one of experimental pain models in rodents, such as the formalin test. To study a relation between these antinociceptive effects with an endogenous opioid system we treated experimental rats with opioid receptor antagonists, a non-selective naloxone and CTOP in the rostral ACC pre- and post-following injections with NSAIDs. CTOP is a short cyclic octapeptide (D-Phe-Cys-Tyr-D-Trp-Orn-Thr-Pen-Thr-$_{NH2}$) that selectively antagonizes with a mu-opioid receptor (MOR).

Antinociceptive Effects of NSAIDs Injected into the ACC

Firstly, we tested the effects of the NSAIDs on thermal and mechanical paw withdrawal reflexes during the post-formalin inflammatory phase (phase II). Five min following intraplantar formalin injection (the phase I), prior to the injection of NSAIDs into the rACC, all animals showed a significant reduction in thermal paw withdrawal latency and mechanical withdrawal threshold compared to pre-baseline values ($p < 0.001$) (Figure 11A, C). These data show some spreading hyperalgesia contralaterally, from the formalin-injected paw to the non-injected paw ($p < 0.05$) (Figure 11B, D).

Fifteen minutes after formalin injection, either saline, diclofenac, ketoprofen, ketorolac or lornoxicam was administered into the rACC, and thermal and mechanical paw withdrawals were assessed again bilaterally 15 and 45 min later (i.e., at minute 30 and 60 post-formalin) during the phase II. As can be seen in the saline treatment group, withdrawals recovered to near pre-formalin baseline levels. A simple comparison of pre-formalin baselines with thermal paw withdrawal latencies and threshold data at minute 30 and 60 post-formalin clearly shows antinociceptive effects of all NSAIDs in both formalin injected ($p < 0.001$) (Figure 11A, C), and not injected paw ($p < 0.001$) (Figure 11B, D).

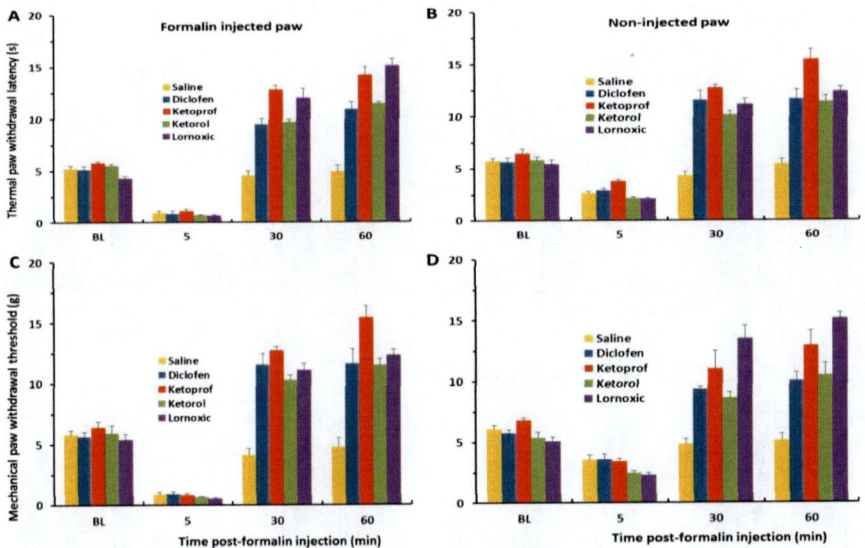

Figure 11. Latencies of the thermal paw withdrawal reflex (s) (A, B) and thresholds of the mechanical paw withdrawal reflex (g) (B, D) after intraplantar formalin injection to one (right) paw. Note analgesics result in a significant increase in latencies and thresholds compared to the saline control for post-formalin phase II (at 30 min and 60 min), in formalin injected (A, C) and non-injected (B, D) paws. BL – pre-formalin baseline.

Pre-Treatment with Naloxone Prevents NSAIDs-Induced Antinociception

In the second set of experiments, we tested if pretreatment with non-selective opioid receptors' antagonist naloxone would prevent NSAIDs-induced antinociception in the rostral area of ACC in the post-formalin phase II. Ten minutes after unilateral intraplantar injection of formalin, rats received naloxone, followed 15 min later by microinjection of one of the NSAIDs, diclofenac, ketorolac, ketoprofen, lornoxicam or saline. Pretreatment with naloxone completely prevented any thermal or mechanical antinociceptive or anti-hyperalgesic effect of all four NSAIDs during the phase II in the formalin-injected paw (Figure 12A, C). In the non-injected paw, we observed almost the same reduction of antinociceptive effects of all NSAIDs in the rACC during the phase II for thermal and mechanical paw withdrawal reflexes (Figure 12B, D).

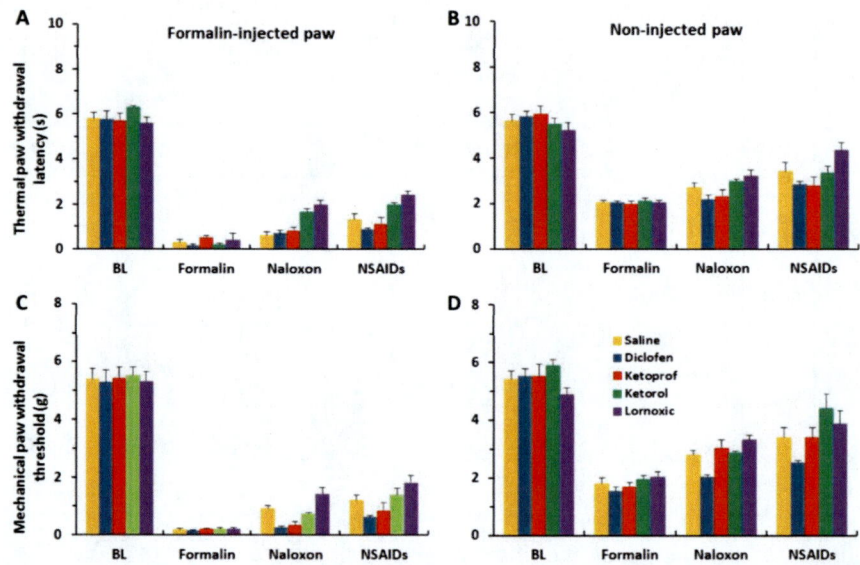

Figure 12. Pretreatment with opioid receptor antagonist naloxone completely prevents analgesic effects of NSAIDs in ipsilateral (formalin injected) paw (A, C) and contralateral (non-injected) paw (B, D) in latencies of the thermal paw withdrawal reflex (s) (A, B) and thresholds of the mechanical paw withdrawal reflex (g) (C, D) for post-formalin phase II (30 min), respectively.

Post-Treatment with Naloxone Abolishes NSAIDs-Induced Antinociception

In the third set of experiments, we tested whether post-treatment with naloxone abolishes NSAIDs-induced antinociception in the rACC at 30 min of post-formalin. These results showed that naloxone abolished thermal or mechanical antinociceptive reactions of all four NSAIDs almost to the baseline level (Figure 13A, C). For the non-injected paw, we observed the same effects of naloxone for all NSAIDs in the rACC during phase II for thermal and mechanical paw withdrawal reflexes (Figure 13B, D).

Pre-Treatment with CTOP Prevents NSAIDs-Induced Antinociception

In the same manner as naloxone, pretreatment with selective MOR antagonist CTOP completely prevented NSAIDs-induced anti-nociception in the rACC in the post-formalin phase II (Figure 14A, C). In the non-injected paw, we observed almost the same reduction of antinociceptive effects of all NSAIDs (Figure 14B, D).

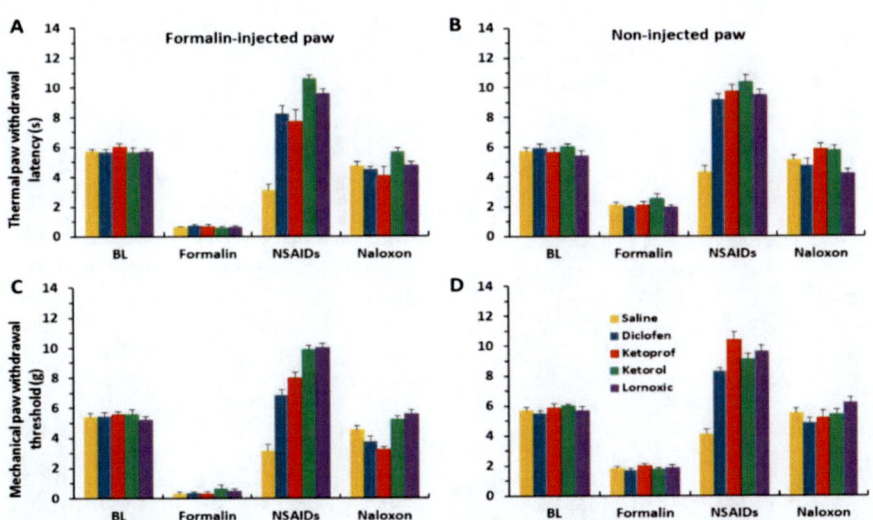

Figure 13. Post-treatment with opioid receptor antagonist naloxone completely abolishes analgesic effects of NSAIDs in ipsilateral (formalin injected) paw (A, C) and contralateral (non-injected) paw (B, D) in latencies of the thermal paw withdrawal reflex (s) (A, B) and thresholds of the mechanical paw withdrawal reflex (g) (C, D) for post-formalin phase II (30 min), respectively.

Post-Treatment with CTOP Abolishes NSAIDs-Induced Antinociception

In the last set of experiments, post-treatment with CTOP followed NSAIDs, also completely abolished analgesia produced by diclofenac, ketoprofen, ketorolac and lornoxicam injected into the rACC (Figure 15A, C). For formalin non-injected paw, we observed almost same reduction of antinociceptive effects of these NSAIDs (Figure 15B, D).

The present findings have shown that microinjection of widely used NSAIDs (diclofenac, ketoprofen, ketorolac and lornoxicam) in the rACC induces antinociception in an inflammatory pain model induced by intraplantar injection of formalin into one (right) hindpaw of rats. These data confirmed our previous results in an acute pain model with TF and HP tests (Gurtskaia et al., 2014a; Tsagareli et al., 2010, 2011, 2012; Tsagareli, Tsiklauri, 2012; Tsiklauri et al., 2016).

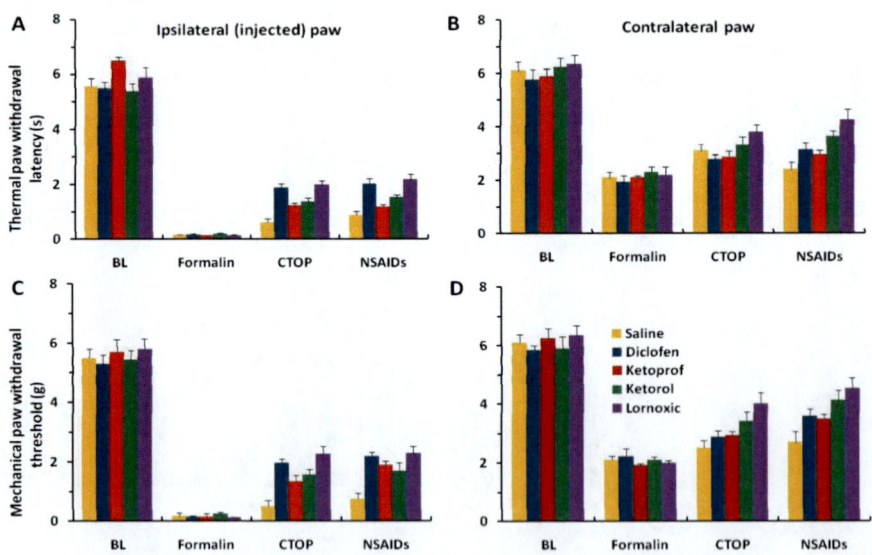

Figure 14. Pretreatment with MOR antagonist CTOP completely prevents analgesic effects of NSAIDs in ipsilateral (formalin injected) paw (A, C) and contralateral (non-injected) paw (B, D) in latencies of the thermal paw withdrawal reflex (s) (A, B) and thresholds of the mechanical paw withdrawal reflex (g) (C, D) for post-formalin phase II (30 min), respectively.

Antinociceptive Tolerance to NSAIDs in Anterior Cingulate Cortex 57

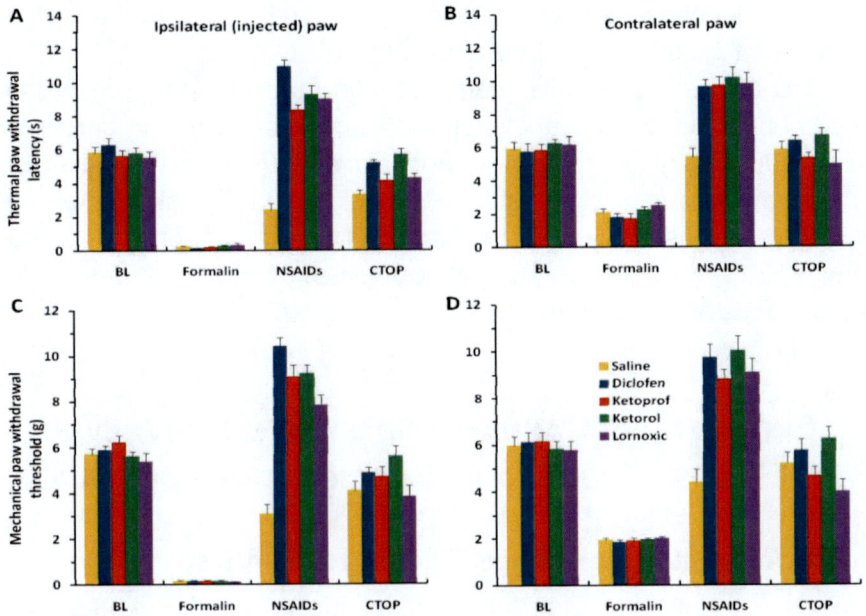

Figure 15. Post-treatment with MOR antagonist CTOP completely abolished analgesic effects of NSAIDs in ipsilateral (formalin injected) paw (A, C) and contralateral (non-injected) paw (B, D) in latencies of the thermal paw withdrawal reflex (s) (A, B) and thresholds of the mechanical paw withdrawal reflex (g) (C, D) for post-formalin phase II (30 min), respectively.

According to the recently established concepts, the mechanism producing NSAIDs analgesia can be due to blocking induction of prostaglandins and of involvement of endogenous opioid peptides (Heinricher, Fields, 2013; Vanegas et al., 2010). We have recently clearly shown that systemic pre-treatment with naloxone completely prevented the analgesic effects of i.p. injected NSAIDs, in thermal paw withdrawal and mechanical paw withdrawal tests in the formalin model of pain (Tsiklauri et al., 2017).

In this study, we have revealed that pre- or post-treatment with naloxone and CTOP injected into the rACC significantly prevented or diminished NSAIDs-induced antinociception. These data support the role for the endogenous opioidergic descending pain control circuits. The latter consists of the brainstem pain modulatory periaqueductal grey (PAG) – rostral ventro-medial medulla (RVM) axis underscoring the strong convergence of antinociceptive mechanisms for non-opioid and opioid analgesics (Heinricher, Fields, 2013; Heinricher, Ingram, 2009; Vanegas et al., 2010; Vazquez et al., 2007).

In conclusions, here we demonstrated that microinjection broadly used non-opioid, NSAID analgesics injected into the rostral part of the ACC, induced significant antinociception in rats. Pre- and post-injections of opioid receptor antagonists, naloxone and CTOP strong reduced NSAIDs analgesic effects. The present findings support the concept that NSAIDs-evoked antinociception is mediated *via* descending endogenous opioid system.

ENDOGENOUS CANNABINOID SYSTEM IS INVOLVED IN NSAIDS – INDUCED ANTINOCICEPTIVE TOLERANCE

Antinociceptive Tolerance Effects to NSAIDs

Apart of opioid mechanisms, the second neuromodulatory system involving in the pathophysiology of pain that has recently recruited a particular interest for the development of new therapeutic strategies is the endocannabinoids system (ECS) that plays a key role in pain control. This system is integrated by the cannabinoid receptors, their endogenous ligands, and the enzymes involved in the synthesis and degradation of these ligands (Di Marzo et al., 2015; Hohman, Rice, 2013; Lau, Vaughan, 2014a; Maldonado et al., 2016). Experimental and clinical studies have shown the importance of the ACC in affective aspects of pain (Craig, 2006). In this work we investigated the brain mechanisms of NSAIDs antinociception in the formalin test for the developing of tolerance. To study a relation these antinociceptive effects with endocannabinoids we treated experimental rats with CB1 receptor antagonist AM-251 in the rACC following injections with diclofenac, ketoprofen, ketorolac, and lornoxicam.

As in a previous investigation, at the first day of this experiment all four NSAIDs, resulted in significant antinociception in the formalin test (Figure 16).

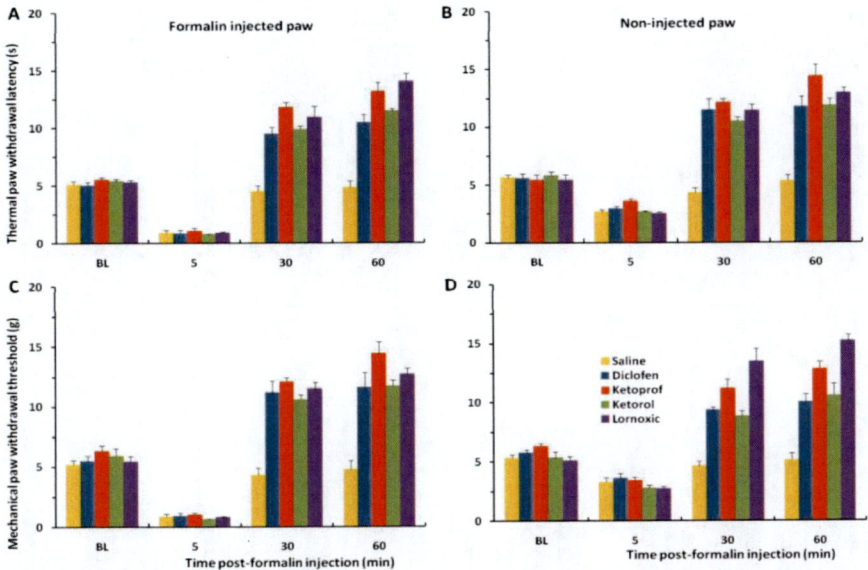

Figure 16. Latencies of the thermal paw withdrawal reflex (s) (A, B) and thresholds of the mechanical paw withdrawal reflex (g) (B, D) after intraplantar formalin injection to one (right) paw at the first day of the experiment. Note analgesics result in a significant increase in latencies and thresholds compared to the saline control for post-formalin phase II (at 30 min and 60 min), in formalin injected (A, C) and non-injected (B, D) paws. BL – pre-formalin baseline.

However, in four consecutive days NSAIDs microinjections into the rACC resulted in progressively less antinociception, so by day 4 there was no effect, that was similar to saline microinjections for both behavioral tests, i.e. induced tolerance. At the last, the fourth day, post-treatment with AM-251 did not change the latency of thermal and threshold of mechanical withdrawal reflexes (Figure 17). This means that the CB1 receptor antagonist does not affect behavioral withdrawal responses in the tolerant rats' group, unlike the rats on the first experimental day (Figure 16).

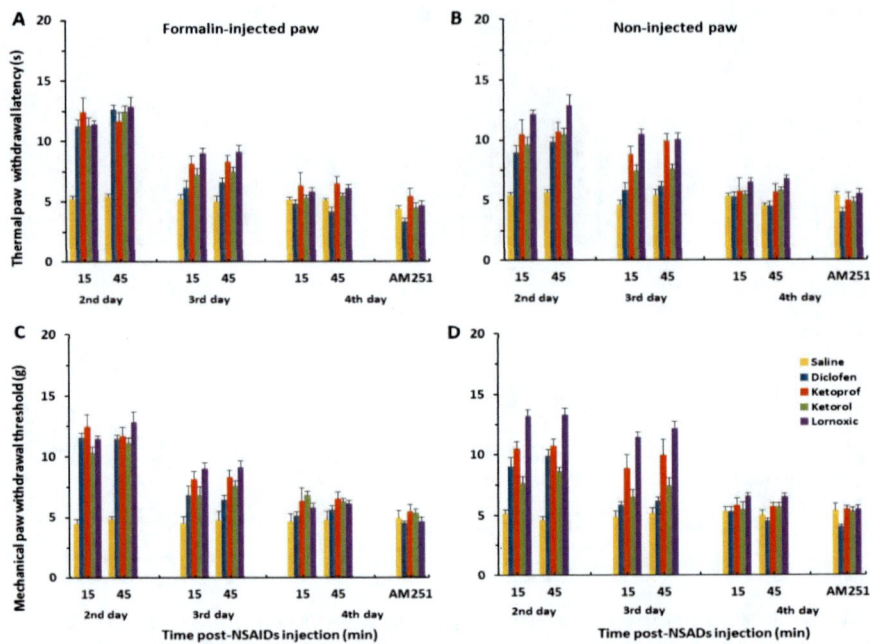

Figure 17. Latencies of the thermal paw withdrawal reflex (s) (A, B) and thresholds of the mechanical paw withdrawal reflex (g) (C, D) after NSAIDs administration into the ACC for three consecutive days. Note in subsequent 2–4 days antinociception decreased gradually for formalin injected (A, C) and non-injected (B, D) paws, respectively, i.e., developed tolerance. Note, at the fourth day, post-treatment with AM-251 does not change the latency of thermal and threshold of mechanical withdrawal reflexes.

Pre- and Post-Treatment with AM-251

In the second set of this study, we tested if pretreatment with AM-251 would prevent NSAIDs-induced antinociception in the rACC in the post-formalin phase II. Ten minutes after unilateral intraplantar injection of formalin, rats received AM-251, followed 15 min later by microinjection of one of the NSAIDs or saline. Pretreatment with AM-251 completely prevented any thermal or mechanical antinociceptive or antihyperalgesic effect of all four NSAIDs during the phase II in the formalin-injected paw (Figure 18A, C). In the non-injected paw, we observed almost same reduction of antinociceptive effects of all NSAIDs in the rACC during phase II for thermal and mechanical paw withdrawal reflexes (Figure 18B, D).

In the last set of experiments, post-treatment with AM-251 followed NSAIDs, almost completely abolished analgesia produced by diclofenac, ketoprofen, ketorolac and lornoxicam injected into the rACC (Figure 19A, C). For formalin non-injected paw, we observed the same reduction of antinociceptive effects of these NSAIDs (Figure 19B, D).

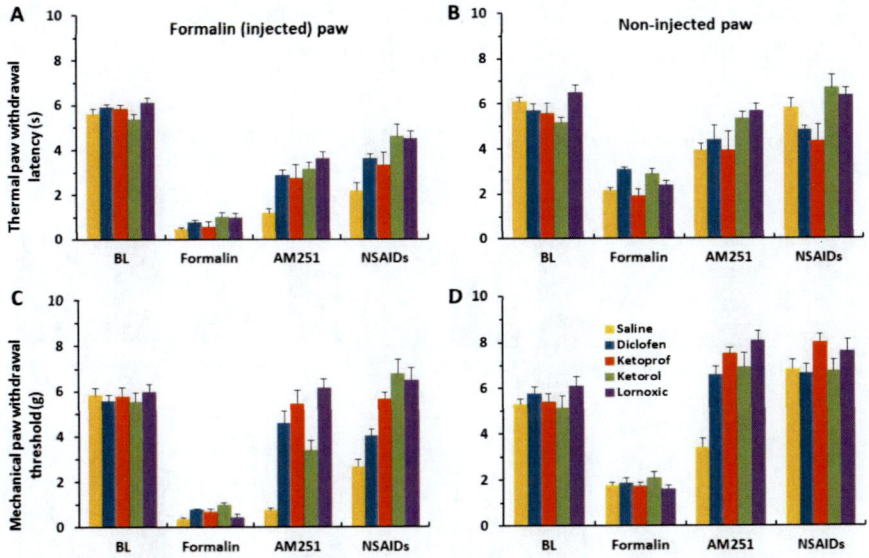

Figure 18. Pretreatment with CB1 receptor antagonist AM-251 completely prevents analgesic effects of NSAIDs in ipsilateral (formalin injected) paw (A, C) and contralateral (non-injected) paw (B, D) in latencies of the thermal paw withdrawal reflex (s) (A, B) and thresholds of the mechanical paw withdrawal reflex (g) (C, D) for post-formalin phase II (30 min), respectively.

According to presented data, CB1 receptor antagonist AM-251 completely prevented the analgesic effects of diclofenac, ketoprofen, ketorolac and lornoxicam in both ipsilateral and contralateral paws. These findings confirm previous evidence where pretreatment with AM-251 either into the lateral-ventro-lateral (LVL) PAG or into the RVM prevented antinoci61aptive effects of metamizole in Carrageenan model of hind paw inflammation of rats (Escobar et al., 2012). As authors concluded, NSAIDs might induce analgesia by acting through three mechanisms in the PAG – RVM axis. Firstly, inhibition of COXs would depress the pro-nociceptive effects caused by prostaglandins *via* the RVM. Secondly, inhibition of prostaglandin synthesis would increase the availability arachidonic acid, whose products decrease synaptic inhibition. Thirdly, by inhibiting the COXs, NSAIDs protect endocannabinoids from degradation and this also decrease synaptic inhibition (Escobar et al., 2012). As we have shown here, in this descending modulatory pathway NSAIDs synergized with endogenous opioids (Gurtskaia et al., 2014a; Tsagareli, Tsiklauri, 2012; Tsagareli et al., 2012; Tsiklauri et al., 2016; 2017; 2018a,b).

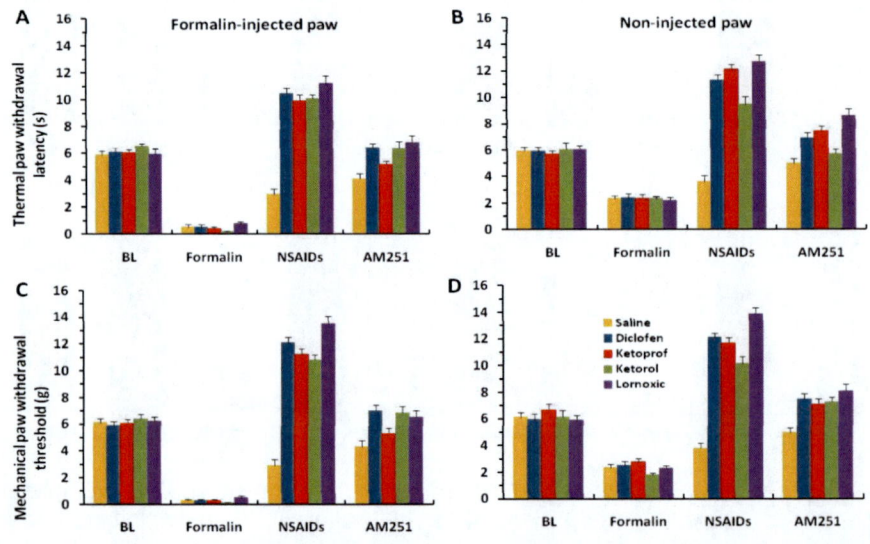

Figure 19. Post-treatment with CB1 receptor antagonist AM-251 completely abolishes analgesic effects of NSAIDs in ipsilateral (formalin injected) paw (A, C) and contralateral (non-injected) paw (B, D) in latencies of the thermal paw withdrawal reflex (s) (A, B) and thresholds of the mechanical paw withdrawal reflex (g) (C, D) for post-formalin phase II (30 min), respectively.

In the PAG–RVM axis, the action NSAIDs is reduced by the CB1 receptor antagonist AM-251. Reduction of gamma-amino butyric acid (GABA) inhibition increases the activity PAG output neurons, which, *via* the RVM cause descending antinociception at the spinal cord level (Escobar et al., 2012). Taken together, these and our results suggest that descending inhibition of nociception triggered at the PAG by non-opioid analgesics, as well as by opioids, cannabinoids, GABA antagonists and other agents, depends at least partly on endocannabinoid-induced and CB1 receptor-mediated decrease in GABAergic inhibition of spinally projecting, pain-inhibiting neurons in the RVM (Escobar et al., 2012; Tsiklauri et al., 2016; Vanegas et al., 2010).

Chapter 6

ANTINOCICEPTIVE TOLERANCE TO NSAIDS IN INSULAR CORTEX

A growing body of literature suggests that the brain region that is a part of the pain processing network, the insula, is both anatomically and functionally well suited to serve a primary and fundamental role in pain processing. By quantitative perfusion neuroimaging to investigate slowly varying neural states highly relevant to a complex phenomenon, such as pain, Segerdahl with coauthors (2015) identified the dorsal posterior insula as subserving a fundamental role in pain and as the likely human homologue of the nociceptive region identified from animal studies. Especially with regard to pain experience, the insular cortex (IC) has been presumed to participate in both sensory-discriminative and affective-motivational aspects of pain (Lu et al., 2016).

The agranular insular cortex (AIC) is found in other mammals including cats, monkeys, primates, and humans as well. In primates, the divisions of the IC are the same as in rats, and the AIC occupies an area immediately noticeable, that is, dorsal to the primary olfactory cortex. The rats AIC is a small region of the cerebral cortex located on the lateral area of the cerebral hemispheres that is involved in the perception and response to pain (Jasmin, Ohara, 2009). Direct injections of morphine into the AIC increase dopamine and GABA levels, resulting in behavioral antinociception (Jasmin et al., 2003). The major connections of the AIC are with areas that have established roles in behavior responses to noxious stimuli. The AIC projections to other cortical areas and subcortical sites such as the amygdala are likely to participate in the sensorimotor integration of nociceptive processing, while the hypothalamus and brainstem projections are most likely to contribute to descending pain inhibitory control (Jasmin, Ohara, 2009).

In the present study, we proposed that the analgesic effects of the three NSAIDs, diclofenac, ketorolac and lornoxicam (xefocam) microinjected into the AIC would exhibit antinociceptive tolerance mediated *via* endogenous opioids. Representative microinjection sites are shown in the Figure 20 (see methodologies in detail, the chapter 8).

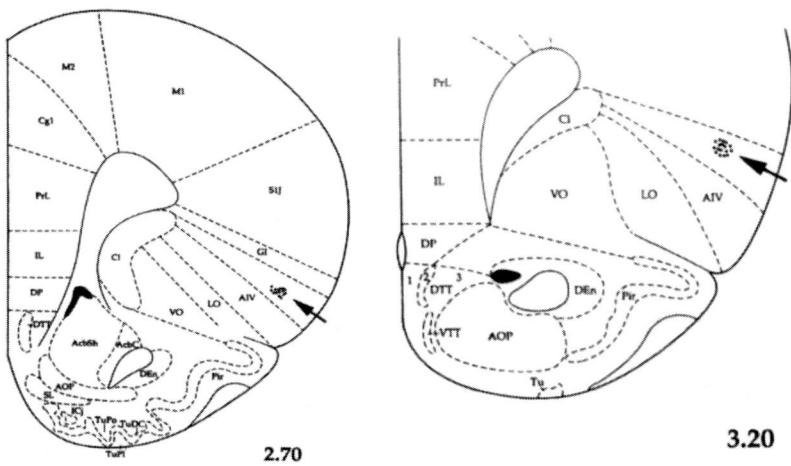

Figure 20. Serial coronal sections of the rat brain showing placement of microinjections in the AIC (black arrows). The number below each section represents millimeters relative to bregma. Adapted from the Stereotaxic atlas in Paxinos G, Watson C. *The Rat Brain in Stereotaxic Coordinates.* Compact third edition. San Diego, CA: Academic Press; 1997.

Tolerance to Antinociceptive Effects of NSAIDs in AIC

In the first set of experiments, we found that microinjection of NSAIDs into the AIC produced antinociception, as revealed by a latency increase in the TF and HP compared to the baseline control of intact rats and a control group with saline microinjected into the same site. The repeated-measures ANOVA revealed that the TF latency significantly increased for diclofenac [$F(9, 20) = 56.229$, $P < 0.0001$], ketorolac [F(9,

20) = 30.398, $P < 0.0001$], and lornoxicam (xefocam) [F(9, 20) = 53.058, $P < 0.0001$], respectively, but not for saline group [F(9,20) = 1.941, $P = 0.1428$, not significant]. On the first experimental day, the differences between NSAIDs-treated groups and the intact control group were significant for diclofenac ($t = 18.549$, $P < 0.001$), for ketorolac ($t = 12.024$, $P < 0.001$), and for lornoxicam ($t = 17.696$, $P < 0.001$), respectively. The TF latency differences between NSAIDs-treated groups and the saline control group by Dunnett's test were significant on the first experimental day for diclofenac ($t = 4.940$, $P < 0.01$), ketorolac ($t = 2.541$, $P < 0.05$), and lornoxicam ($t = 5.733$, $P < 0.01$), respectively (Figure 21A).

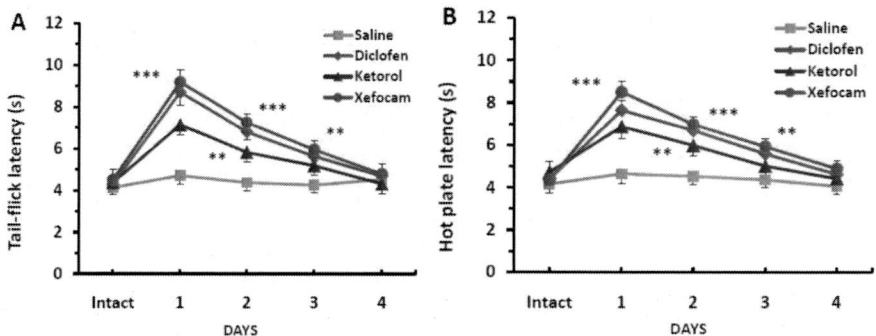

Figure 21. Microinjections of NSAIDs into the AIC for 4 consecutive days. (A) A progressive decrease in TF latency as compared to intact control group; (B) a progressive decrease in HP latency to intact control group. Statistical analysis was performed by repeated-measure ANOVA with post hoc Tukey–Kramer's multiple comparisons test; n=6 per test group; **-$P < 0.01$, ***-$P < 0.001$.

We found similar significant differences of enhancement in the HP latencies compared to the intact group for diclofenac [F(9, 20) = 51.749, $P < 0.0001$], for ketorolac [F(9,20) = 43.359, $P < 0.0001$], and for lornoxicam [F(9,20) = 38.551, $P < 0.0001$], respectively, but not for saline control [F(9,20) = 2.681, $P = 0.0613$, not significant]. Here also on the first experimental day, the differences between NSAIDs-treated groups and the intact control group were significant for diclofenac ($t = 16.989$, $P < 0.001$), ketorolac ($t = 14.209$, $P < 0.001$), and lornoxicam ($t = 15.488$, $P < 0.001$), respectively (Figure 21B). The HP latency differences between NSAIDs-treated groups and the saline control group by Dunnett's test were significant in the first experimental day for diclofenac ($t = 6.938$, $P < 0.01$), for ketorolac ($t = 5.012$, $P < 0.01$), and for xefocam ($t = 7.580$, $P < 0.01$).

Subsequent NSAIDs microinjections into the AIC caused gradually less antinociception, so by day 4 there was no effect, that was similar to saline microinjections for both the TF and the HP tests, i.e. induced tolerance (Figure 21A, B). On the second experimental day, the TF latency differences between NSAIDs-treated groups and the saline control group by Dunnett's test were significant for lornoxicam ($t = 4.065$, $P < 0.01$) and diclofenac ($t = 3.090$, $P < 0.05$), but not for ketorolac ($t = 0.9749$, $P > 0.05$, not significant). On the third and fourth experimental days, there were no significant differences between NSAID-treated groups and the saline control (Figure 21A).

Concerning the HP test, on the second experimental day, the latency differences between NSAIDs-treated groups and the saline group by Dunnett's test were significant for diclofenac ($t = 4.534$, $P < 0.01$), lornoxicam ($t = 4.576$, $P < 0.01$), and ketorolac ($t = 2.899$, $P < 0.05$), respectively. On the third day, there were significant differences for xefocam ($t = 3.345$, $P < 0.01$) and diclofenac ($t = 3.002$, $P < 0.05$), but not for ketorolac ($t = 1.598$, $P > 0.05$, not significant), while on the fourth day there were no significant differences for any of the NSAIDs (Figure 21B).

Pre-Treatment with Naloxone Prevents NSAIDS-Induced Antinociception

In the second set of experiments, we tested if pretreatment with a nonselective opioid receptor antagonist naloxone prevents antinociception induced by NSAID microinjections into the AIC. Pretreatment with naloxone completely prevented the analgesic effects of diclofenac, ketorolac, and lornoxicam (xefocam) in the TF test. The ANOVA did not reveal significant differences between naloxone injected and NSAIDs-injected groups for diclofenac [$F(2,15) = 0.6083$, $P = 0.2552$, not significant], ketorolac [$F(2,15) = 0.8998$, $P = 0.4275$, not significant], and xefocam [$F(2,15)=3.078$, $P = 0.0758$, not significant], respectively, and hence the TF latencies of the saline, naloxone, and

NSAIDs groups were not significantly different when compared with the post hoc test ($P > 0.05$) (Figure 22A, C, E).

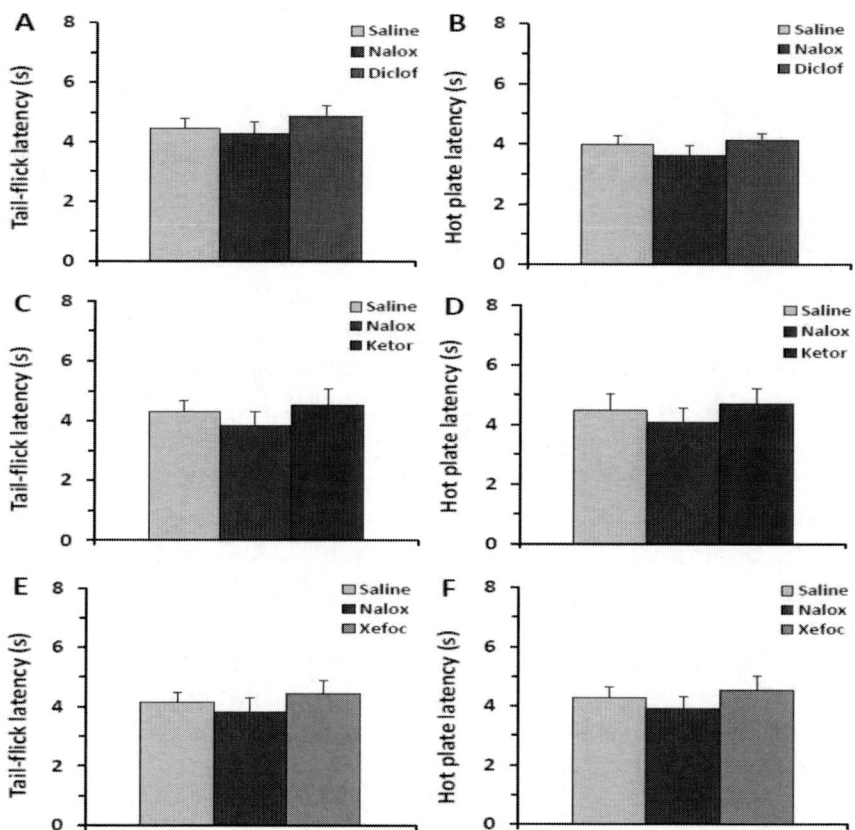

Figure 22. Pretreatment with naloxone before microinjections of NSAIDs into the AIC. (A, C and E) Naloxone prevents NSAID-induced antinociception in TF latency for diclofenac (A), ketorolac (C), and xefocam (E), respectively. (B, D and F) Naloxone prevents NSAID-induced antinociception in HP latency for diclofenac (B), ketorolac (D), and xefocam (F), respectively. Statistical analysis was performed by one-way ANOVA with post hoc Tukey–Kramer's multiple comparisons test; n=6 per test group.

Similar results were observed in the HP test for diclofenac [$F(2,15) = 0.8492$, $P = 0.4473$, not significant], for ketorolac [$F(2,15) = 0.3815$, $P = 0.6893$, not significant], and for xefocam [$F(2,15) = 0.6152$, $P = 0.5536$, not significant], respectively, and hence the HP latencies of the saline, naloxone, and NSAIDs groups were not significantly different when compared with the post hoc test ($P > 0.05$) (Figure 22B, D, F).

Post-Treatment with Naloxone Abolishes NSAIDs-Induced Antinociception

In the third set of experiments, we tested if post-treatment with naloxone abolishes antinociception induced by NSAID microinjections into the AIC. We found that post-treatment with naloxone completely abolished the analgesic effects of diclofenac, ketorolac and lornoxicam in the TF test. The ANOVA revealed significant differences in the TF latencies between saline, NSAIDs, and naloxone groups for diclofenac [$F(2,15) = 87.881$, $P < 0.0001$], for ketorolac [$F(2,15) = 89.175$, $P < 0.0001$], and for xefocam [$F(2,15) = 93.530$, $P < 0.0001$], respectively. Naloxone completely abolished antinociceptive effects of diclofenac ($t = 15.914$, $P < 0.001$), ketorolac ($t = 17.417$, $P < 0.001$), and xefocam ($t = 15.157$, $P < 0.001$), respectively (Figure 23A, C, E). Similar results we obtained in the HP test. Here also, the ANOVA revealed significant differences in the HP latencies between saline, NSAIDs, and naloxone groups for diclofenac [$F(2,15) = 86.529$, $P < 0.0001$], ketorolac [$F(2,15) = 39.425$, $P < 0.0001$], and xefocam [$F(2,15) = 114.22$, $P < 0.0001$], respectively. Opioid antagonist naloxone completely abolished analgesic effects of diclofenac ($t = 15.503$, $P < 0.001$), ketorolac ($t = 11.679$, $P < 0.001$), and xefocam ($t = 17.022$, $P < 0.001$), respectively (Figure 23B, D, F).

The present data have demonstrated that microinjections of diclofenac, ketorolac and lornoxicam, into the AIC induce antinociception. These results are similar to the findings of previous investigations in an acute pain model with TF and HP tests, and in which metamizole, xefocam, ketorolac or lysine-acetylsalicylate were given systemically or microinjected into the PAG, the CeA and the NRM (Pernia-Andrade et al., 2004; Tortorici, Vanegas, 2000; Tortorici et al., 2009; Tsagareli, Tsiklauri, 2012; Tsagareli et al., 2010, 2011; Tsiklauri et al., 2010, 2016; Vanegas, Tortorici, 2007). In another study, responses of spinal dorsal horn wide-dynamic range neurons to mechanical noxious stimulation in hindpaw of rats were strongly inhibited by intravenous metamizole (Telleria-Diaz et al., 2010). Moreover, repeated microinjections of these NSAIDs into the AIC over a period of 4 days resulted in development of tolerance due to a progressive decrease in antinociceptive effectiveness, reminiscent of that usually induced by opiates (Tortorici et al., 2003, 2004; Tsagareli, Tsiklauri, 2012; Tsiklauri et al., 2010). These findings confirm our previous results in which development of tolerance was observed to the analgesic effects of diclofenac, ketorolac and xefocam microinjected into the DH of rats. After administration of each NSAID, a progressive decrease in the TF and HP latency (i.e., tolerance) was noticed over the 4-day period (Gurtskaia et al., 2014a; Tsiklauri et al., 2016). According to the recently established conception or notion, the mechanism producing tolerance to NSAIDs can be due to involvement of endogenous opioid peptides (Tsagareli, Tsiklauri, 2012; Vanegas et al., 2010; Heinricher, Fields, 2013; Heinricher, Ingram, 2009). In this study, we have clearly shown that pre- and post-treatment of a nonselective opioid receptor antagonist naloxone significantly diminishes NSAIDs-induced antinociception. These findings confirm our previous evidence where NSAIDs antinociception in the DH was reduced by pre- as well as post-treatments with naloxone (Gurtskaia et al., 2014a; Tsiklauri et al., 2016). We have just recently showed that systemic pretreatment with naloxone completely prevented the analgesic effects of i.p. injected NSAIDs, in thermal paw withdrawal and mechanical paw withdrawal tests in the formalin model of pain (Tsiklauri et al., 2017).

All presented data confirm the other results that antinociception induced by systemic metamizole involves endogenous opioids that can be blocked by naloxone at the levels of the PAG, the NRM and the spinal dorsal horn, as well as findings that endogenous opioids are involved in the potentiation of analgesia observed with a combination of morphine plus dipyrone (Hernandez-Delgadillo, Cruz, 2006; Vazquez et al., 2005). These data support a role for endogenous opioidergic descending pain-control circuits. The latter consists of the brainstem pain modulatory PAG–RVM medulla axis underscoring the strong convergence of antinociceptive mechanisms for non-opioid and opioid analgesics (Tortorici et al., 2009; Vanegas et al., 2010; Heinricher, Fields, 2013; Heinricher, Ingram, 2009; Vazquez et al., 2007).

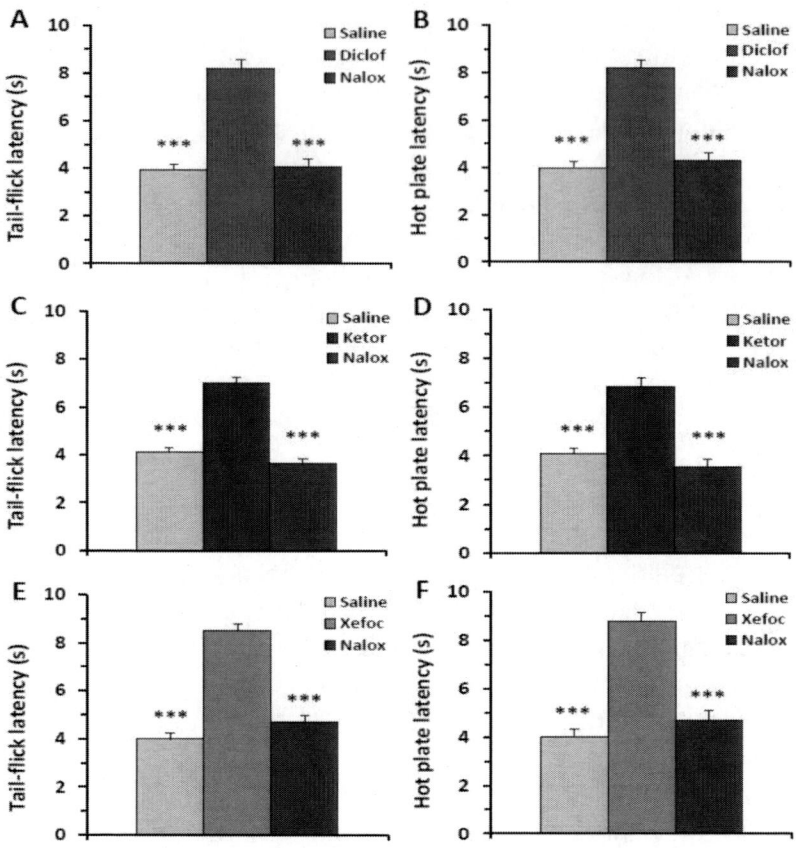

Figure 23. Post-treatment with naloxone (0.2 μg/0.5 μL) after microinjections of NSAIDs into the AIC. (A, C and E) Naloxone abolishes NSAID-induced antinociception in TF latency for diclofenac (A), ketorolac (C), and xefocam (D), respectively. (B, D and F) Naloxone abolishes NSAID-induced antinociception in HP latency for diclofenac (B), ketorolac (D), and xefocam (F), respectively. Each NSAID-injected group shows significant difference vs saline control and vs naloxone post-treated groups in both tests. Statistical analysis was performed by one-way ANOVA with post hoc Tukey–Kramer's multiple comparisons test; n = 6/group. ***$P < 0.001$.

In summary, we showed here for the first time that microinjections of diclofenac, ketorolac, and lornoxicam into the AIC, induce antinociception in male rats. Repeated administration leads to tolerance development to these drugs. The present data support the notion that the development of tolerance to the antinociceptive effects of NSAIDs is mediated *via* an endogenous opioid system, possibly involving descending pain modulatory circuits.

ENDOGENOUS OPIOID SYSTEM IS INVOLVED IN NSAIDS – INDUCED ANTINOCICEPTION

In these experiments we tested an involvement of opioid receptors in NSAIDs-induced antinociception in the AIC using the formalin test. We treated experimental rats with mu-opioid receptor antagonists, CTOP and nonselective naloxone in the AIC pre- and post-following injections with NSAIDs, diclofenac, ketoprofen, ketorolac, and lornoxicam by the Hargreaves and von Frey tests.

NSAIDs-Induced Antinociception and Post-Treatment Effects of CTOP in the AIC

In this first series, we tested the effects of the NSAIDs on thermal and mechanical paw withdrawal reflexes during the post-formalin phase II, at 30 min. Firstly, five min following intraplantar formalin injection (phase I), prior to the injection of NSAIDs into the AIC, all animals showed a very strong reduction in thermal paw withdrawal latency and mechanical withdrawal threshold compared to pre-baseline values ($p < 0.001$) (Figure 24A, C). The ANOVA revealed significant differences in the thermal paw withdrawal latencies between saline, NSAIDs, and CTOP groups for diclofenac [$F(7,40) = 146.71$, $P < 0.0001$], for ketoprofen [$F(7,32) = 133.99$, $P < 0.0001$], for ketorolac [$F(7,40) = 84.812$, $P < 0.0001$], and for lornoxicam [$F(7,40) = 104.28$, $P < 0.0001$], respectively. CTOP significantly reduced antinociceptive effects of diclofenac ($t = 15.754$, $P < 0.001$), ketoprofen ($t = 18.255$, $P < 0.001$), ketorolac ($t = 7.322$, $P < 0.001$), and lornoxicam ($t = 15.769$, $P < 0.001$), respectively (Figure 24A). There are corresponding effects in the contralateral, formalin non-injected paw ($P < 0.001$) (Figure 24B).

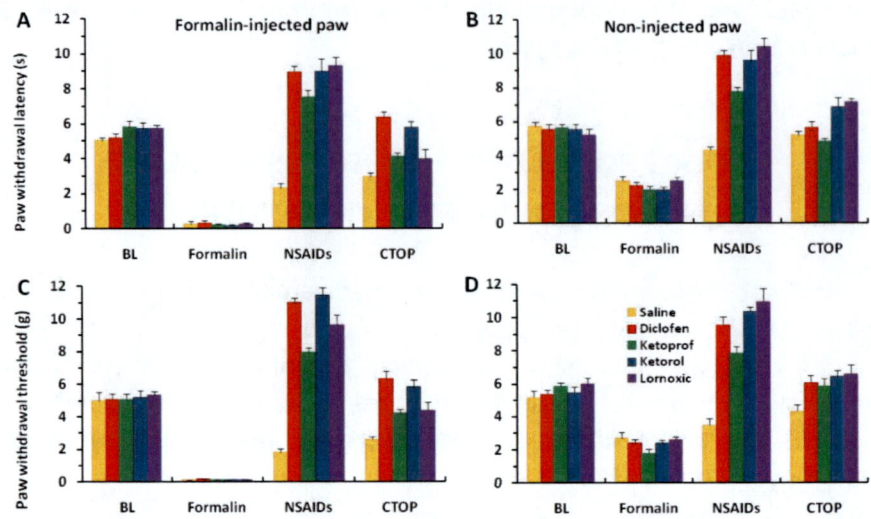

Figure 24. NSAIDs-induced antinociception, and post-treatment with mu-opioid receptor antagonist CTOP results in abolish analgesic effects of NSAIDs in ipsilateral (formalin injected) paw (A, C) and contralateral (non-injected) paw (B, D) in latencies of the thermal paw withdrawal reflex (s) (A, B) and thresholds of the mechanical paw withdrawal reflex (g) (C, D) for post-formalin phase II (30 min), respectively.

Similar results we founded in the mechanical paw withdrawal threshold test (Figure 24C, D). The ANOVA revealed significant differences in the thresholds between saline, NSAIDs, and CTOP groups for diclofenac [$F_{(7,40)}$ = 94.362, $P < 0.0001$], ketoprofen [$F_{(7,32)}$ = 80.206, $P < 0.0001$], ketorolac [$F_{(7,40)}$ = 118.45, $P < 0.0001$], and lornoxicam [$F_{(7,40)}$ = 57.358, $P < 0.0001$], respectively. Selective MOR antagonist CTOP reduced analgesic effects of diclofenac ($t = 13.054$, $P < 0.001$), ketoprofen ($t = 12.189$, $P < 0.001$), ketorolac ($t = 16.618$, $P < 0.001$), and lornoxicam ($t = 11.212$, $P < 0.001$), respectively (Figure 24C). There was significant spreading hyperalgesia compare to baseline values, and then analgesia, following CTOP antinociceptive effects tested in the non-injected paw ($p < 0.001$) (Figure 24D).

Pre-Treatment with CTOP Prevents NSAIDs-Induced Antinociception

In the second session of this study, pretreatment with the selective MOR antagonist CTOP prevented NSAIDs-induced antinociception in the AIC for the post-formalin phase II in both thermal and mechanical tests (Figure 25A, C). In the contralateral paw we observed almost the same reduction of antinociceptive effects of all NSAIDs (Figure 25B, D).

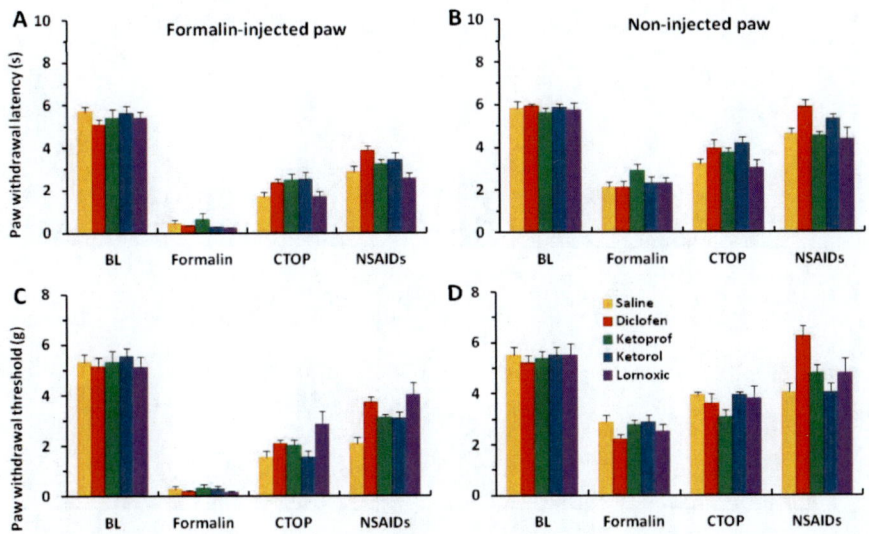

Figure 25. Pretreatment with MOR antagonist CTOP prevents analgesic effects of NSAIDs in ipsilateral (A, C) and contralateral (non-injected) paw (B, D) in latencies of the thermal paw withdrawal reflex (s) (A, B) and thresholds of the mechanical paw withdrawal reflex (g) (C, D) for post-formalin phase II (30 min), respectively.

Here, there were not significant differences between CTOP treated and NSAIDs treated rat groups for ketoprofen (t=2.536, $P > 0.05$), ketorolac ($t = 3.239$, $P > 0.05$), and lornoxicam ($t = 2.69$, $P > 0.05$), respectively, but not for diclofenac ($t = 5.54$, $P < 0.05$), in Hargreaves test (Figure 25A). There were almost the same trend effects for the non-formalin injected paw in all analgesics except in diclofenac ($t = 6.705$) ($p < 0.01$) (Figure 25B). Similar results we obtained in the von Frey test for ketoprofen ($t = 3.364$, $P > 0.05$), ketorolac ($t = 3.994$, $P > 0.05$), and lornoxicam ($t = 2.453$, $P > 0.05$), respectively, but not for diclofenac ($t = 5.72$, $P < 0.05$) (Figure 25C). There were the same trend effects in the contralateral paw, again except for diclofenac ($t = 8.62$, $P < 0.001$) (Figure 25D).

Pre-Treatment with Naloxone Prevents NSAIDs-Induced Antinociception in AIC

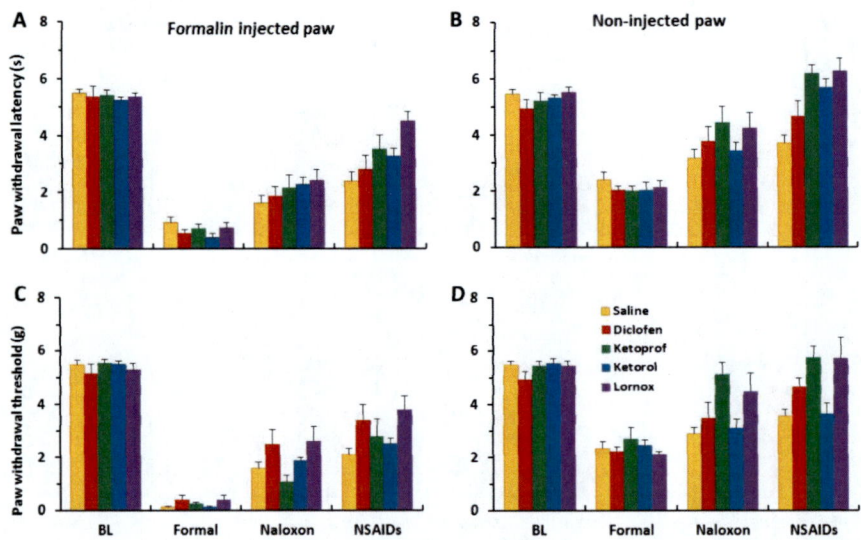

Figure 26. Pretreatment with opioid antagonist naloxone prevents analgesic effects of NSAIDs in ipsilateral (formalin injected) paw (A, C) and contralateral (non-injected) paw (B, D) in latencies of the thermal paw withdrawal reflex (s) (A, B) and thresholds of the mechanical paw withdrawal reflex (g) (C, D) for post-formalin phase II (30 min), respectively.

In the third session of this study, we investigated whether pretreatment with naloxone prevented NSAIDs-induced antinociception in the AIC in the post-formalin phase II in both thermal and mechanical behavioral tests (Figure 26). Here, blocking effects of naloxone were similar to CTOP effects in the previous experimental session.

In particular, there were not significant differences between naloxone treated and NSAIDs treated groups of rats for diclofenac ($t = 2.288$, $P > 0.05$), for ketoprofen ($t = 3.912$, $P > 0.05$), for ketorolac ($t = 2.11$, $P >$

0.05), respectively, but not for lornoxicam ($t = 4.69$, $P < 0.05$), in the thermal test (Figure 26A). There were almost the same effects for the non-formalin injected paw in all analgesics except in lornoxicam ($t = 6.816$) ($p < 0.01$) (Figure 26B). Similar results we observed in the mechanical pressing test for diclofenac ($t = 1.87$, $P < 0.05$), ketoprofen ($t = 3.713$, $P > 0.05$), ketorolac ($t = 3.283$, $P > 0.05$), and for lornoxicam ($t = 2.369$, $P > 0.05$), respectively (Figure 26C). There were the same effects in the non-formalin injected paw ($P > 0.05$) (Figure 26D).

Post-Treatment with Naloxone Abolishes NSAIDs-Induced Antinociception in AIC

In this fourth session, the ANOVA revealed significant differences in the thermal paw withdrawal latencies between saline, NSAIDs, and naloxone groups for diclofenac [$F(7,40) = 80.667$, $P < 0.0001$], for ketoprofen [$F(7,32) = 89.08$, $P < 0.0001$], for ketorolac [$F(7,40) = 93.29$, $P < 0.0001$], and for lornoxicam [$F(7,40) = 102.67$, $P < 0.0001$], respectively. Naloxone significantly abolished antinociceptive effects of diclofenac ($t = 14.815$, $P < 0.001$), ketoprofen ($t = 13.586$, $P < 0.001$), ketorolac ($t = 17.789$, $P < 0.001$), and lornoxicam ($t = 15.329$, $P < 0.001$), respectively (Figure 27A). There are corresponding effects in the formalin non-injected paw ($P < 0.001$) (Figure 27B).

Similar results were obtained in the mechanical paw withdrawal threshold test (Figure 27C, D). The ANOVA revealed significant differences in the thresholds between saline, NSAIDs, and naloxone groups for diclofenac [$F(7,40) = 82.706$, $P < 0.0001$], ketoprofen [$F(7,32) = 80.665$, $P < 0.0001$], ketorolac [$F(7,40) = 86.131$, $P < 0.0001$], and lornoxicam [$F(7,40) = 115.63$, $P < 0.0001$], respectively. Naloxone reduced analgesic effects of diclofenac ($t = 15.619$, $P < 0.001$), ketoprofen ($t = 17.209$, $P < 0.001$), ketorolac ($t = 11.038$, $P < 0.001$), and lornoxicam ($t = 21.775$, $P < 0.001$), respectively (Figure 27C). There was significant spreading hyperalgesia compare to baseline values, and then analgesia, following naloxone anti-nociceptive effects tested in the formalin non-injected paw ($P < 0.001$) (Figure 27D).

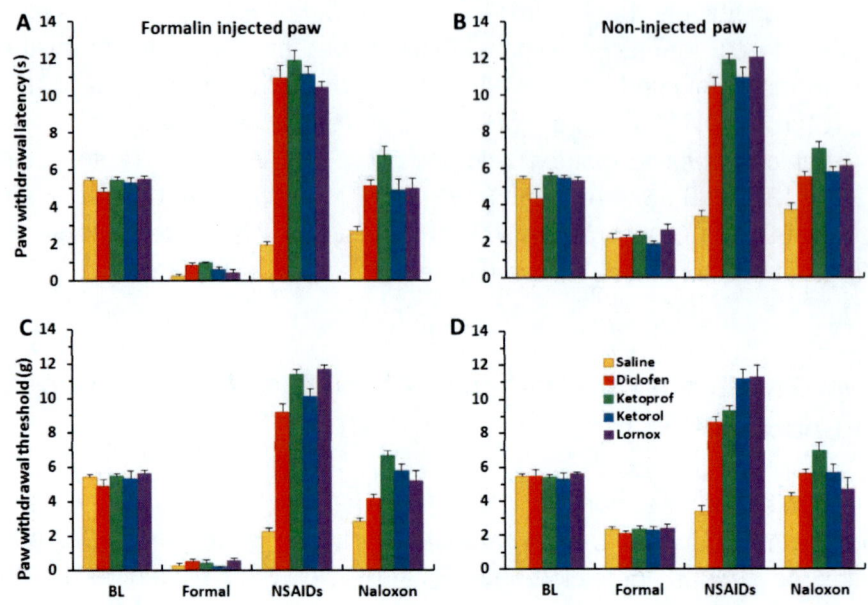

Figure 27. NSAIDs-induced antinociception, and post-treatment with opioid receptor antagonist naloxone results in abolish analgesic effects of NSAIDs in ipsilateral (formalin injected) paw (A, C) and contralateral (non-injected) paw (B, D) in latencies of the thermal paw withdrawal reflex (s) (A, B) and thresholds of the mechanical paw withdrawal reflex (g) (C, D), respectively for post-formalin phase II (30 min).

ENDOGENOUS CANNABINOID SYSTEM IS INVOLVED IN NSAIDS – INDUCED ANTINOCICEPTION

To study a relation of antinociceptive effects of NSAIDs with endocannabinoids we treated experimental rats with CB1 receptor antagonist AM-251 in the AIC following injections with diclofenac, ketoprofen, ketorolac, and lornoxicam.

Pre-Treatment with AM-251

In this set of this study, we tested if pretreatment with AM-251 would prevent NSAIDs-induced antinociception in the AIC in the post-formalin phase II. Ten minutes after unilateral intraplantar injection of formalin, rats received AM-251, followed 15 min later by microinjection of one of the NSAIDs or saline. Pretreatment with AM-251completely prevented any thermal and mechanical paw withdrawal antinociceptive effects of all four NSAIDs in the formalin-injected paw (Figure 28A, C).

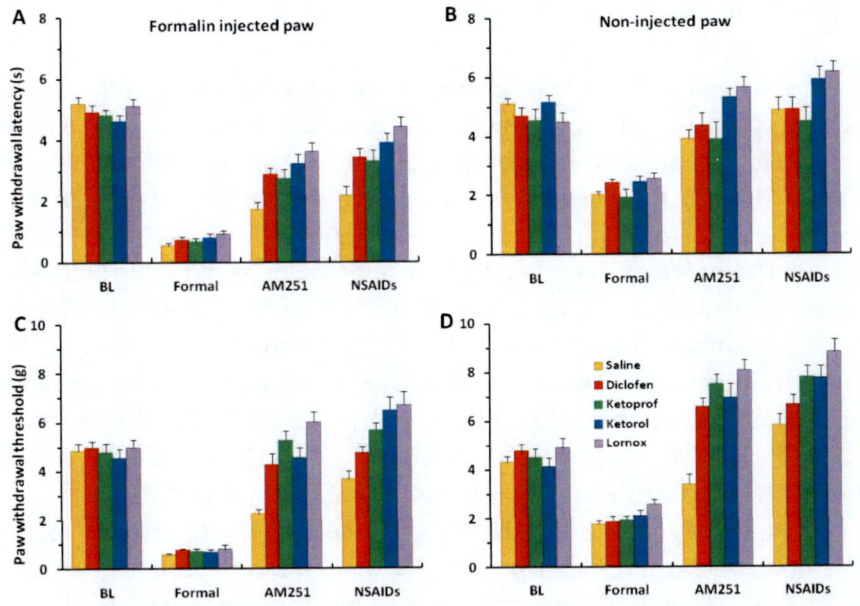

Figure 28. Pretreatment with CB1 receptor antagonist AM-251 prevents analgesic effects of NSAIDs in ipsilateral (A, C) and contralateral hindpaws (B, D) in thermal latencies (s) (A, B) and thresholds (g) of paw withdrawals (C, D), respectively.

Bonferroni Multiple Comparison Test of selected pairs of columns revealed non-significant values for diclofenac (t = 1.259, P > 0.05), ketoprofen (t = 1.305, P > 0.05), ketorolac (t = 1.534, P > 0.05), and lornoxicam (t = 1.824, P > 0.05) in the Hargreaves test (Figure 28A), and of in von Frey test for diclofenac (t = 0.7264, P > 0.05), ketoprofen (t = 0.6585, P > 0.05), lornoxicam (t = 1.102, P > 0.05), but not for ketorolac (t = 3.192, P < 0.05, significant) (Figure 28C). In the formalin non-injected paw we observed almost the same non-significant reduction of antinociceptive effects of all NSAIDs in the thermal test for diclofenac (t = 0.9415, P > 0.05), ketoprofen (t = 1.041, P > 0.05), ketorolac (t = 1.029, P > 0.05), and lornoxicam (t = 0.8891, P > 0.05) (Figure 28B), and also in the mechanical test for diclofenac (t = 1.035, P > 0.05), ketoprofen (t = 0.4293, P > 0.05), ketorolac (t = 1.266, P > 0.05), and lornoxicam (t = 1.130, P > 0.05) (Figure 28D).

Post-Treatment with AM-251

In the final set of these experiments, post-treatment with AM-251 followed NSAIDs, almost completely abolished analgesia produced by diclofenac, ketoprofen, ketorolac and lornoxicam injected into the AIC (Figure 29A, C). In the Hargreaves test, the difference between NSAIDs and AM-251 injected groups is significant [ANOVA, $F(7,40) = 22.652$, $P < 0.0001$]. Bonferroni post-hoc test for selected pairs revealed significant values for diclofenac (t = 5.694, P < 0.001), ketoprofen (t = 6.890, P < 0.001), ketorolac (t = 6.161, P < 0.001), and lornoxicam (t = 6.264, P < 0.001) (Figure 29A). In the contralateral paw we observed the same reductions of antinociceptive effects of these NSAIDs for diclofenac (t = 6.259, P < 0.001), ketoprofen (t = 5.869, P < 0.001), ketorolac (t = 5.583, P < 0.001), and lornoxicam (t = 5.964, P < 0.001) (Figure 29B).

In von Frey test, the ANOVA revealed significant value for the differences between NSAIDs and AM-251 injected groups [$F(7,40) = 31.712$, $P < 0.0001$]. Bonferroni post-hoc test for selected pairs gave out significant values for diclofenac (t = 7.062, P < 0.001), ketoprofen (t = 6.521, P < 0.001), ketorolac (t = 7.367, P < 0.001), and lornoxicam (t = 8.325, P < 0.001) (Figure 29C). Similar effects of paw withdrawal threshold reduction we found in the contralateral paw for diclofenac (t = 6.056, P < 0.001), ketoprofen (t = 5.793, P < 0.001), ketorolac (t = 6.003, P < 0.001), and lornoxicam (t = 5.898, P < 0.001) (Figure 29D).

The present findings have shown that microinjection of commonly used NSAIDs (diclofenac, ketoprofen, ketorolac and lornoxicam) in the AIC produced antinociception in an inflammatory pain model induced by intraplantar injection of formalin into one hindpaw of rats. These results confirmed our evidence in an acute pain model with TF and HP tests. These data also confirmed our previous findings obtained in other pain matrix structures, such as the central nucleus of amygdala (Tsagareli et al., 2009), the nucleus raphe magnus (Tsagareli et al., 2011), periaqueductal grey (Tsagareli et al., 2012), dorsal hippocampus (Gurtskaia et al., 2014), and anterior cingulate cortex (Tsiklauri et al., 2018).

Some spreading hyperalgesic or analgesic effects from the ipsi- into the contralateral paw that we observed in this study are explained as to be due to central sensitization or desensitization at the spinal cord level. We suppose that in these experiments such sensitization/ desensitization can activate or inhibit the system of commissural interneurons that is present in spinal cord and brainstem and which can develop some formalin-induce hyperalgesia or NSAIDs-induced analgesia. This phenomenon is well-documented in pain medicine (see review, Koltzenburg et al., 1999).

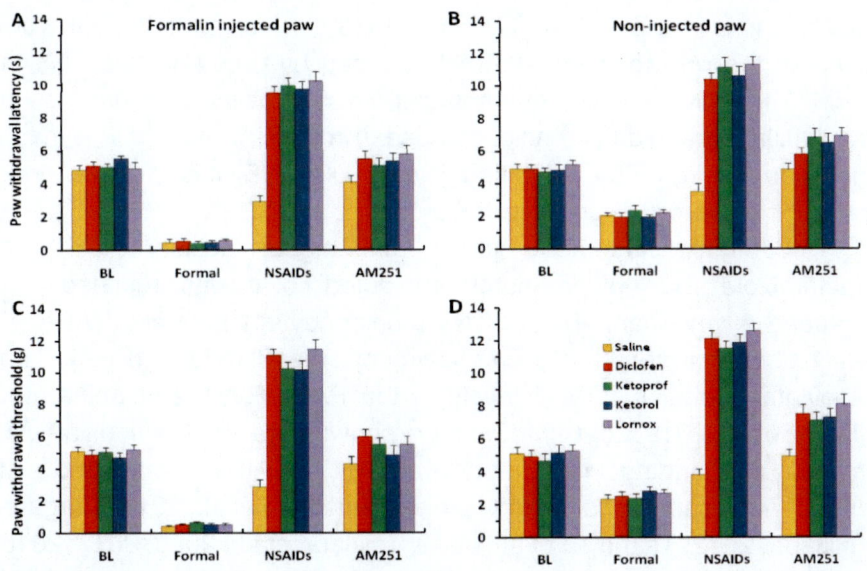

Figure 29. Post-treatment with AM-251 results in abolish analgesic effects of NSAIDs in ipsilateral (A, C) and contralateral paws (B, D) in withdrawal latencies (s) (A, B) and thresholds (g) (C, D), respectively.

Here we have revealed that pre- or post-treatment with naloxone and CTOP injected into the AIC significantly prevented or diminished NSAIDs-induced antinociception. These data support the role of the endogenous opioidergic descending pain control circuits. The latter consists of the brainstem pain modulatory periaqueductal grey (PAG)–rostral ventro-medial medulla (RVM) axis underscoring the strong convergence of antinociceptive mechanisms for non-opioid and opioid analgesics (Chen, Heinricher, 2019; Heinricher, Fields, 2013; Vanegas et al., 2010; Vazquez et al., 2007).

According to presented data, the CB1 receptor antagonist AM-251 completely prevented or attenuated the analgesic effects of diclofenac, ketoprofen, ketorolac and lornoxicam in both ipsilateral and contralateral paws. These findings confirm previous evidence where pretreatment with AM-251 either into the lateral-ventro-lateral PAG or into the RVM reduced antinociceptive effects of metamizole in Carrageenan model of hindpaw inflammation of rats (Escobar et al., 2012). As these authors concluded, NSAIDs might induce analgesia by acting through three mechanisms in the PAG–RVM axis. Firstly, inhibition of COXs would depress the pro-nociceptive effects caused by prostaglandins *via* the RVM. Secondly, inhibition of prostaglandin synthesis would increase the availability arachidonic acid, whose products decrease synaptic inhibition. Thirdly, by inhibiting the COXs, NSAIDs protect endo-cannabinoids from degradation (Escobar et al., 2012).

Recently it has been found that higher doses of dipyrone (metamizole), but not paracetamol injected i.p. in rats, resulted in an increase of endocannabinoids [N-arachidonoylethanolamide (AEA), 2-arachidonoyl-glycerol (2-AG), palmitoylethanolamide (PEA), and oleoylethanolamide (OEA)] levels in the PAG, RVM, and spinal cord (Topuz et al., 2019; 2020). As we have shown here and previous articles, in this descending modulatory pathway NSAIDs synergized with endogenous cannabinoids and opioids (Gurtskaia et al., 2014; Tsagareli, Tsiklauri, 2012; Tsagareli et al., 2012; Tsiklauri et al., 2016; 2017; 2018).

In the PAG–RVM axis, the action NSAIDs is reduced by the CB1 receptor antagonist AM-251. Reduction of GABA inhibition increases the activity PAG output neurons, which, *via* the RVM cause descending antinociception at the spinal cord level (Escobar et al., 2012). Taken together, these results suggest that descending inhibition of nociception triggered at the PAG by non-opioid analgesics, as well as by opioids, cannabinoids, GABA antagonists, depends at least partly on endocannabinoid-induced and CB1 receptor-mediated decrease in GABA-ergic inhibition of spinally projecting, pain-inhibiting neurons in the RVM (Escobar et al., 2012; Tsiklauri et al., 2016; Vanegas et al., 2010).

Overall, here we demonstrated that microinjection widely used non-opioid analgesics, such as diclofenac, ketoprofen, ketorolac and lornoxicam injected into the AIC, induced significant antinociception in rats. Pre- and post-injections of opioid receptor antagonists, naloxone and CTOP as well as CB1 receptor antagonist AM-251 resulted in a strong reduction NSAIDs analgesic effects in both ipsilateral and contralateral paws. These data support the concept that NSAIDs-evoked antinociception is mediated *via* descending endogenous opioid and cannabinoid systems inhibiting spinal withdrawal reflexes in rodents.

As stated above, the AIC is a portion of the insula that lies in the anterior part of the central sulcus in humans. The anterior insula is divided into two sub-regions: an agranular region of the ventral anterior insula and a dysgranular region of the dorsal anterior to middle insular cortex. In general, the dysgranular area is gustatory cortex, whereas the agranular area is proposed to be involved in the regulation of physiological changes associated with emotional states, including noxious emotional experience. In rodents, the IC is a portion of the cerebral cortex folded deeply within the lateral sulcus surrounding the rhinal fissure – hidden by the frontal and temporal opercula (Jasmin, Ohara, 2009). This cytoarchitecture of the IC corresponds with its connectivity patterns and functions in an internal disassociation in pain processing. The posterior IC (PIC) participates in the somatosensory features of pain, while the anterior cortical portion preferably mediates its affective aspects (Craig, 2011; Lu et al., 2016).

Some evidence from animal, preclinical, and clinical studies suggests that the IC is involved in both the sensory and affective dimensions of pain. Particularly, in the shaping of pain perception, the AI serves as a critical site where multimodal information competes and integrates with nociception to create an awareness of the body state. The progression to chronic pain reflects not only impairment of the normal functional activity of the insula, but also the disruption of specific circuits that modulate pain-related emotional awareness involving the IC (Craig, 2011; Jasmin, Ohara, 2009; Lu et al., 2016).

It is likely that plastic changes involving glutamatergic receptors touch off the onset of pain chronification, and subsequent pERK (protein kinase RNA-like endoplasmic reticulum kinase) signaling pathways underpin the abnormal activation of the pain-processing system through dysfunction of pain-modulating receptors such as GABA-ergic and dopaminergic receptors (Ohara et al., 2003; Qui et al., 2013, 2014). Besides, although most studies propose involvement of the AIC and PIC in isolated functional networks of pain, as there are intimate reciprocal links between anterior and posterior areas, evidence on functional interactions within the insula is imperative for a deeper insight into the role of the insula in pain (Lu et al., 2016).

In conclusions, as pain is a complex perception in which sensation, emotion, and cognition interweave, conscious perception and the unpleasantness of pain are mirrored by behavioral reactions (e.g. withdrawal reactions, escape or sweating due to suffering), which require activity in wide brain regions. Our study clearly showed that antinociceptive tolerance effects in the AIC are mediated by opioid and cannabinoid mechanisms and pain experience in the formalin test arouse behavioral responses and activate the descending pain modulatory system.

Chapter 7

NSAIDs–INDUCED ANTINOCICEPTION IN CENTRAL NUCLEUS OF AMYGDALA

Studies of the emotional and motivational basis of pain reveal a diverse and complex set of processes by which the affective experience of pain is realized. Negative emotions concomitant pain can exacerbate chronic pain. The amygdala with its well-documented role in emotion processing and related disorders, such as anxiety, depression, and persistent pain, strongly supports the concept that the amygdala is a key player in the emotional modulation of chronic pain. The central nucleus of amygdala (CeA) are particularly important for sensory and emotion processing, and is now defined as the "nociceptive amygdala" because of its high content of nociceptive neurons, receiving specific pain information directly from the spino-parabrachio-amygdaloid pain pathway (Baliki, Apkarian, 2015; Craig, 2006; Keay, Bandler, 2009; Neugebauer, 2015; Seymour, Dolan, 2013).

The long period required for chronic pain to be established might correspond to the period demanded for the time-dependent plastic changes and their consolidation in the central pain network underlying this sensory and emotional experience. Of the "pain matrix' structures, the plastic changes in the connection from the parabrachial nucleus to the central amygdala are of particular interest because the CeA, one of the major targets of the projections from the lateral parabrachial nucleus (LPB), plays essential roles in emotional memory and responses and is also a site for innate and learned fear/threat against aversive events, making it likely that this is the pathway playing a central role in the "emotional" aspect of pain (Kato et al., 2018).

Here we report the role of endogenous opioid and cannabinoid receptors in modulation of pain by injection their antagonists into the CeA and PAG (see methodologies in detail, the chapter 8).

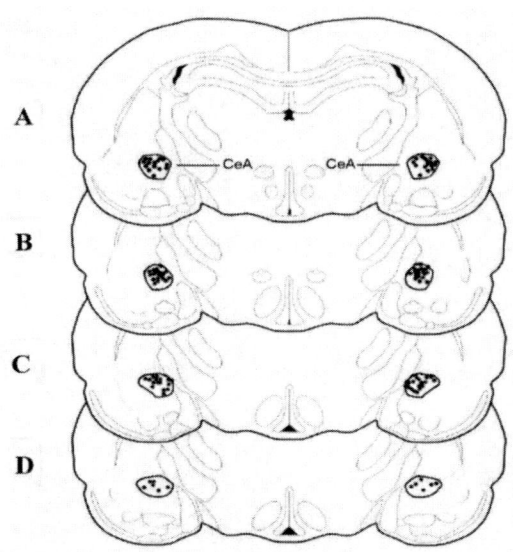

Figure 30. Serial coronal sections of the rat brain showing placement of microinjections of NSAIDs or saline in CeA (filled circles) simplified from Paxinos & Watson's atlas (1997). The distances from the interaural line ±4.3 mm and from the bregma is –2.12 mm (A), –2.30 mm (B), –2.56 mm (C), and –2.80 mm (D), respectively.

ANTINOCICEPTIVE EFFECTS OF NSAIDS INJECTED INTO CENTRAL AMYGDALA IS ATTENUATED BY COMBINED ADMINISTRATION OF OPIOID AND CANNABINOID RECEPTOR ANTAGONISTS

In our previous work we clearly showed antinociceptive tolerance to NSADs in the CeA (Tsagareli et al., 2010; 2012). Here we report that this antinociception is mediated *via* endogenous opioid and cannabinoid systems in the formalin model of pain. In the first set of these experiments, five min following intraplantar formalin injection all animals showed a significant reduction in thermal paw withdrawal latency and mechanical withdrawal threshold compared to pre-baseline values. Fifteen minutes after formalin injection, NSAIDs injected into the CeA (microinjection sites are shown in the Figure 30) clearly showed antinociceptive effects of withdrawal behavioral reactions in rats (Figure 31).

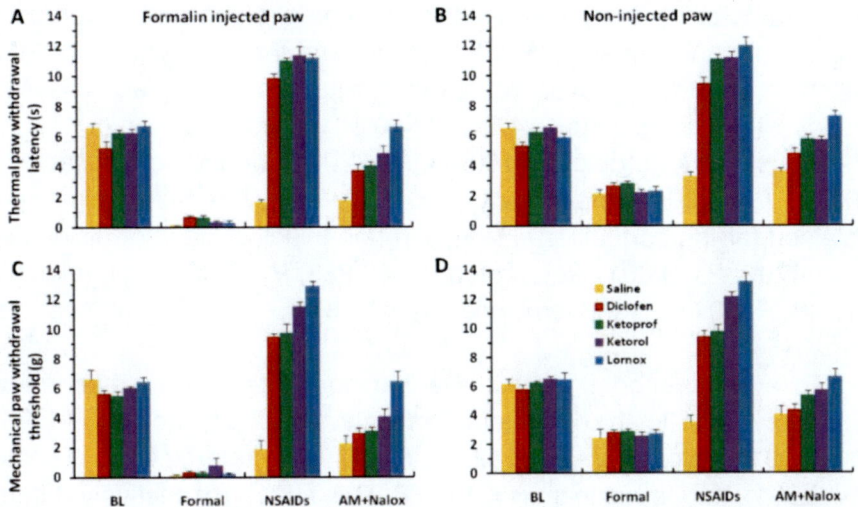

Figure 31. Post-treatment with a combined CB1 receptor antagonist AM-251 and naloxone significantly reduces analgesic effects of NSAIDs in ipsilateral (formalin injected) paw (A, C) and contralateral (non-injected) paw (B, D) in latencies of the thermal paw withdrawal (s) (A, B) and thresholds of the mechanical paw withdrawal (g) reflexes (C, D), respectively for post-formalin phase II (30 min).

Post-Treatment with a Combined AM-251 and Naloxone in CeA

When we post-treated with a combined cannabinoid CB1 receptor antagonist AM-251 and opioid receptors antagonist naloxone, we found a significant abolish of analgesic effects of NSAIDs, diclofenac, ketoprofen, ketorolac and lornoxicam (Figure 31).

In the thermal test, ANOVA revealed significant values for the treated groups with diclofenac [F(7,40) = 62.616, $P < 0.0001$], with ketoprofen [F(7,40) = 80.102, $P < 0.0001$], with ketorolac [F(7,40) = 96.283, $P < 0.0001$], and with lornoxicam [F(7,40) = 84.801, $P < 0.0001$], respectively. Similar effects we found in the mechanical (von Frey) test with diclofenac [F(7,40) = 73.914, $P < 0.0001$], ketoprofen [F(7,40) = 84.425, $P < 0.0001$], ketorolac [F(7,40) = 83.857, $P < 0.0001$], and lornoxicam [F(7,40) = 84.801, $P < 0.0001$], respectively. Post-hoc Tukey-Kramer Multiple Comparisons Test revealed significant differences between mean values in NSAIDs injected and then in a combined AM-251 plus naloxone treated groups in the ipsilateral (formalin injected) hindpaw for diclofenac (t = 14.515, $P < 0.001$), for ketoprofen (t = 16.48, $P < 0.001$), for ketorolac (t = 15.339, $P < 0.001$), and for lornoxicam (t = 10.912, $P < 0.001$), respectively (Fig. 31A). The same differences were obtained for the contralateral (formalin non-injected) paw for diclofenac (t = 11.709, $P < 0.001$), ketoprofen (t = 13.285, $P < 0.001$), ketorolac (t = 14.515, $P < 0.001$), and lornoxicam (t = 11.879, $P < 0.001$), respectively (Fig. 31B).

Tukey-Kramer post hoc test revealed more differences in mechanical (von Frey) test in the ipsilateral hindpaw for diclofenac (t = 14.402, $P < 0.001$), ketoprofen (t = 14.534, $P < 0.001$), ketorolac (t = 16.324, $P < 0.001$), and lornoxicam (t = 14.138, $P < 0.001$), respectively (Figure 31C). Almost the same mean values differences were revealed in the contralateral hindpaw for diclofenac (t = 10.909, $P < 0.001$), ketoprofen (t = 9.543, $P < 0.001$), ketorolac (t = 13.982, $P < 0.001$), and lornoxicam (t = 14.184, $P < 0.001$), respectively (Figure 31D).

Pre-Treatment with a Combined AM-251 and Naloxone in CeA

Pre-treatment with these two combined antagonists resulted in significant reduction NSAIDs-induced antinociception ($P < 0.001$) (Figure 32). Here we also revealed significant ANOVA values for the treated groups with diclofenac [F(7,40) = 82.255, $P < 0.0001$], ketoprofen [F(7,40) = 117.45, $P < 0.0001$], ketorolac [F(7,40) = 107.55, $P < 0.0001$], and lornoxicam [F(7,40) = 109.41, $P < 0.0001$], respectively, in the thermal withdrawals. In the mechanical pressing test similar significant values were found with diclofenac [F(7,40) = 106.29, $P < 0.0001$], ketoprofen [F(7,40) = 89.052, $P < 0.0001$], ketorolac [F(7,40) = 112.9, $P < 0.0001$], and lornoxicam [F(7,40) = 91.719, $P < 0.0001$], respectively.

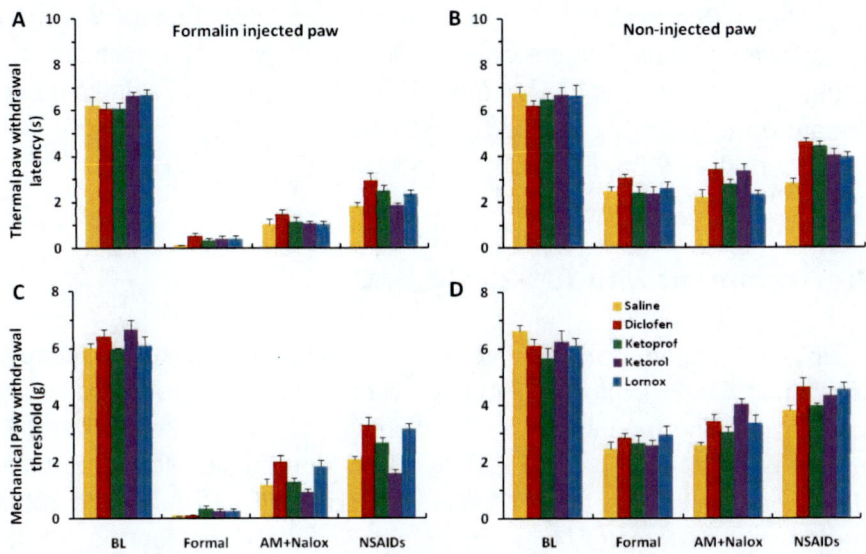

Figure 32. Pre-treatment with a combined CB1 receptor antagonist AM-251 and naloxone in CeA significantly prevents analgesic effects of NSAIDs in ipsilateral (formalin injected) paw (A, C) and contralateral (non-injected) paw (B, D) in latencies of the thermal paw withdrawal reflex (s) (A, B) and thresholds of the mechanical paw withdrawal reflex (g) (C, D), respectively for post-formalin phase II (30 min).

Tukey-Kramer post hoc test revealed not strong but significant differences between mean values of a combined AM-251 plus naloxone treated following NSAIDs injected rats groups in the Hargreaves test for diclofenac (t = 6.703, $P < 0.001$), for ketoprofen (t = 6.146, $P < 0.01$), and for lornoxicam (t = 5.933, $P < 0.01$), but not for ketorolac (t = 3.455, $P > 0.05$), respectively (Figure 32A). Almost the same differences were revealed in the contralateral hindpaw for diclofenac (t = 4.803, $P < 0.05$), ketoprofen (t = 6.688, $P < 0.001$), and for lornoxicam (t = 6.579, $P < 0.001$), but again not for ketorolac (t = 2.744, $P > 0.05$), respectively (Figure 32B).

In the von Frey mechanical withdrawal test Tukey-Kramer post hoc analyze revealed similar differences between pretreatment with AM-251 plus naloxone compare to NSAIDs injected groups for diclofenac ($t = 6.099$, $P < 0.01$), ketoprofen ($t = 6.539$, $P < 0.001$), lornoxicam ($t = 6.255$, $P < 0.01$), but not significant for ketorolac group ($t = 3.08$, $P > 0.05$), respectively (Figure 32C). Some different effects were observed in the contralateral hindpaw where only for diclofenac, the difference of mean values was significant ($t = 4.526$, $P < 0.05$), but not significant for ketoprofen ($t = 3.567$, $P > 0.05$), ketorolac ($t = 1.151$, $P > 0.05$), and lornoxicam ($t = 4.488$, $P > 0.05$), respectively (Figure 32D).

Pre-Treatment with AM-251 in PAG

In the second part of this research, we injected CB1 receptor antagonist AM-251 into the PAG, as the latter is a crucial structure for pain descending modulatory mechanisms of spinal reflexes. When pretreated with AM-251 into the PAG we also found a significant reduction of antinociceptive effects of NSAIDs injected into the CeA (Figure 33). In the thermal test, ANOVA revealed significant values for the treated groups with diclofenac [$F(7,40) = 88.763$, $P < 0.0001$], ketoprofen [$F(7,40) = 76.234$, $P < 0.0001$], ketorolac [$F(7,40) = 87.989$, $P < 0.0001$], and with lornoxicam [$F(7,40) = 78.293$, $P < 0.0001$], respectively.

Tukey-Kramer post-hoc test revealed that differences between AM-251 groups and NSAIDs were not significant for diclofenac ($t = 4.336$, $P > 0.05$) and ketoprofen ($t = 4.168$, $P > 0.05$), but not for ketorolac ($t = 4.548$, $p < 0.05$), and more for lornoxicam ($t = 7.61$, $p < 0.001$) (Figure 33A). These differences were more significant for the contralateral (formalin non-injected) paw for diclofenac ($t = 6.303$, $P < 0.01$), ketorolac ($t = 6.419$, $P < 0.01$), and lornoxicam ($t = 9.303$, $P < 0.001$), but not for ketoprofen ($t = 3.772$, $P > 0.05$) (Figure 33B).

In the von Frey test ANOVA revealed significant values for the treated groups with diclofenac [$F(7,40) = 79.455$, $P < 0.0001$], ketoprofen [$F(7,40) = 89.149$, $P < 0.0001$], ketorolac [$F(7,40) = 78.024$, $P < 0.0001$], and lornoxicam [$F(7,40) = 77.488$, $P < 0.0001$], respectively. Post hoc Tukey-Kramer multiple comparison test revealed the non-significant differences between mean values of CB1 receptor antagonist AM-251 and NSAIDs for ketoprofen (t = 4.493, $P > 0.05$) and for ketorolac (t = 4.493, $P > 0.05$), but not for diclofenac (t = 5.66, $P < 0.01$) and lornoxicam (t = 6.917, $P < 0.001$) (Figure 33C). Almost the same differences were observed for the contralateral paw for diclofenac (t = 6.517, $P < 0.01$) and ketoprofen (t = 6.923, $P < 0.01$), but not for ketorolac (t = 4.216, $P > 0.05$), and lornoxicam (t = 4.361, $P > 0.05$), respectively (Figure 33D).

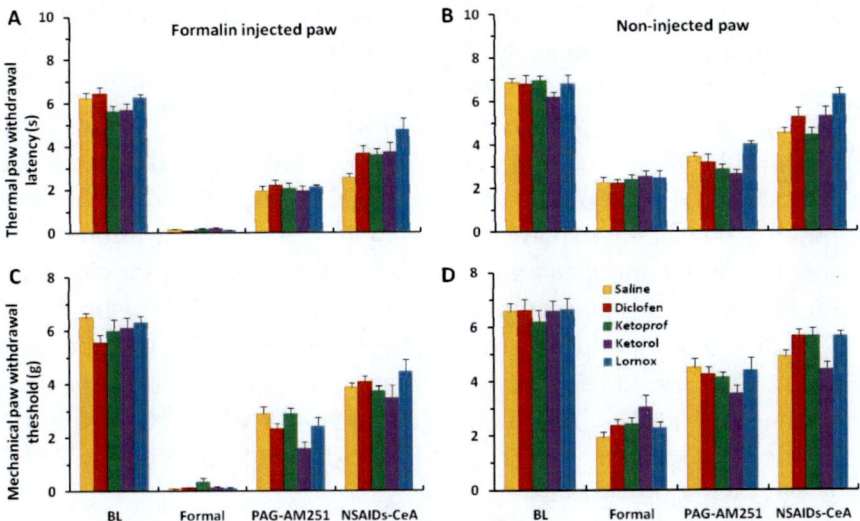

Figure 33. Pre-treatment with CB1 receptor antagonist AM-251 into the PAG significantly prevents analgesic effects of NSAIDs injected into CeA in ipsilateral (formalin injected) paw (A, C) and contralateral (non-injected) paw (B, D) in latencies of the thermal paw withdrawal reflex (s) (A, B) and thresholds of the mechanical paw withdrawal reflex (g) (C, D), respectively for post-formalin phase II (30 min).

Post-Treatment with AM-251 in PAG

In the experiments on post-treated with AM-251 into the PAG we also found a significant reduction of antinociceptive effects of NSAIDs injected into the CeA (Figure 34). In the Hargreaves test, ANOVA revealed significant values for the treated groups with diclofenac [$F(7,40) = 85.523, P < 0.0001$], ketoprofen [$F(7,40) = 154.43, P < 0.0001$], ketorolac [F(7,40) = 102.1, $P < 0.0001$], and lornoxicam [F(7,40) = 123.76, $P < 0.0001$], respectively. Here post-injection of AM-251 is more effective in reduction of NSAIDs-induced antinociception for diclofenac (t = 8.222, $P < 0.001$), ketoprofen (t = 12.746, $P < 0.001$), ketorolac (t = 8.85, $P < 0.001$), and lornoxicam (t = 12.542, $P < 0.001$), respectively (Figure 34A). Similar effects of reduction were observed in the contralateral paw for diclofenac (t = 10.682, $P < 0.001$), ketoprofen (t = 13.898, $P < 0.001$), ketorolac (t = 8.176, $P < 0.001$), lornoxicam (t = 12.47, $P < 0.001$), respectively (Figure 34B).

In the von Frey test ANOVA revealed significant values for the treated groups with diclofenac [F(7,40) = 97.402, $P < 0.0001$], ketoprofen [F(7,40) = 111.12, $P < 0.0001$], ketorolac [F(7,40) = 134.98, $P < 0.0001$], and lornoxicam [F(7,40) = 82.954, $P < 0.0001$], respectively. Differences of mean values between NSAIDs and AM-251 showing reduction of antinociception in the ipsilateral hindpaw were significant for diclofenac (t = 8.293, $P < 0.001$), ketoprofen (t = 10.813, $P < 0.001$), ketorolac (t = 11.769, $P < 0.001$), and lornoxicam (t = 10.04, $P < 0.001$), respectively (Figure 34C). Similar reductions were found in the contralateral paw for diclofenac (t = 11.098, $P < 0.001$), ketoprofen (t = 12.564, $P < 0.001$), ketorolac (t = 11.936, $P < 0.001$), and lornoxicam (t = 10.352, $P < 0.001$), respectively (Figure 34D).

The present data have demonstrated that microinjections of widely used NSAIDs, diclofenac, ketoprofen, ketorolac, and lornoxicam into the CeA resulted in antinociception in the formalin test model of rats. These data are similar to and confirmed our previous tail-flick and hot plate tests in which metamizole (analgin), ketorolac or lornoxicam (xefocam) were given systemically, or microinjected into the CeA, the PAG, or the nucleus raphe magnus (NRM) (Gurtskaia et al., 2014a,b; Tsagareli, Tsiklauri, 2012; Tsagareli et al., 2012; Tsiklauri et al., 2016, 2017, 2018a,b). Pre-treatment or post-treatment with a combination of CB1 antagonist AM-251 and naloxone significantly attenuated NSAIDs antinociception. It is interesting that injections of AM-251 into the PAG also clearly show attenuation of NSAIDs-induced antinociception administered into the CeA. These data strictly confirmed, once more, importance role of the PAG in endocannabinoid modulation of pain. Here we cannot affirm that a combination of AM-251 and naloxone result in cumulative effects on NSAIDs-induced antinociception in the CeA, as both antagonist concentrations are high and the same as in previous experiments.

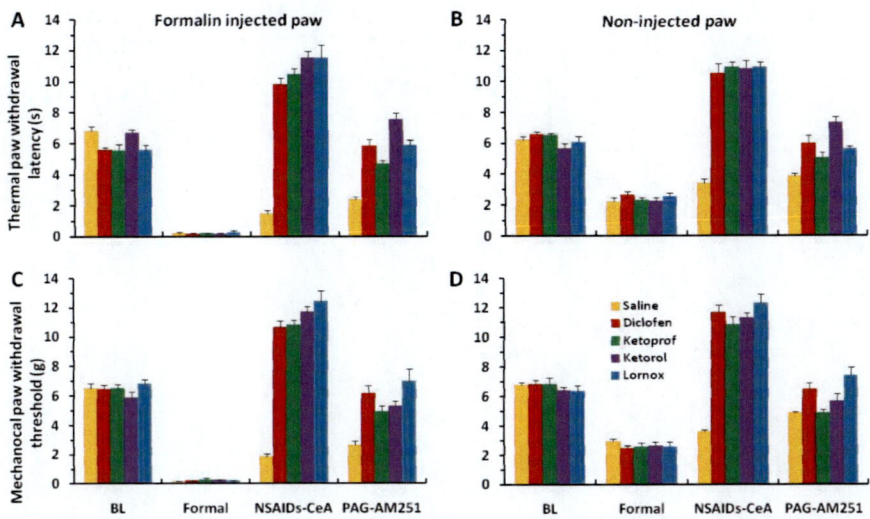

Figure 34. Post-treatment with CB1 receptor antagonist AM-251 into the PAG significantly abolishes analgesic effects of NSAIDs injected into CeA in ipsilateral (formalin injected) paw (A, C) and contralateral (non-injected) paw (B, D) in latencies of the thermal paw withdrawal reflex (s) (A, B) and thresholds of the mechanical paw withdrawal reflex (g) (C, D), respectively for post-formalin phase II (30 min).

Overall, the present findings support the concept that NSAIDs-induced antinociception is mediated *via* descending endogenous opioid and cannabinoid modulatory systems with the central position of the PAG.

Chapter 8

GENERAL DISCUSSION

Presented data clearly showed that pain matrix structures of the limbic brain, responsible for emotional aspects of pain, antinociception, and antinociceptive tolerance to NSAIDs are mediated *via* central opioid and cannabinoid descending modulatory systems controlling spinal nociceptive withdrawal reflexes. Our findings indicated the important role of opioid and cannabinoid receptors in these processes since pre- or post-microinjections of opioid receptors antagonists, naloxone and CTOP, as well as the antagonist CB1 receptor, AM-251 in these brain areas, the ACC, AIC and CeA, significantly prevented or abolished antinociceptive actions of NSAIDs.

CENTRAL ANALGESIC EFFECTS OF NSAIDS

Non-steroidal anti-inflammatory drugs (NSAIDs) are widely prescribed for a variety of painful conditions, and are the backbone in first-line pain management worldwide (Cryer et al., 2016). Their analgesic efficacy has been mainly explained by their peripheral effect in the setting of an inflammatory response to injury. Tissue damage is associated with the release of inflammatory mediators, leading to sensitization of peripheral nociceptors and thus causing sustained pain and hypersensitivity.

Inhibition of the COX-1 and COX-2 by NSAIDs reduces the inflammatory response by inhibiting prostaglandin synthesis, thereby alleviating pain. The COX-2 selective inhibitors (Coxibs) were designed to reduce gastrointestinal side effects associated with conventional NSAIDs (Vuilleumier et al., 2018). In the early 1990's, evidence suggested for the first time that NSAIDs might exert an effect in the CNS, as intrathecally administered NSAIDs were able to abolish hyperalgesia caused by spinal excitatory neuro-transmitters (Malmberg, Yaksh, 1992; Seibert, et al., 1994).

Prostaglandins regulate immune responses, and they are key mediators of pain and other sickness symptoms. In particular, prostaglandin E2 (PGE2) is a key mediator of pain because it sensitizes peripheral and spinal nociceptive pathways. Hence the most common pain treatment is the inhibition of prostaglandin synthesis by cyclooxygenase inhibitors (Natura et al., 2013).

COX-1 is constitutively expressed in peripheral tissues such as gastric mucosa, kidneys or blood platelets, whereas COX-2 is induced in various tissues during inflammatory processes. However, both isoforms are usually present in the CNS. Upon nociceptive stimulation, COX catalyzes the rate-limiting step in prostaglandin synthesis by forming PGH_2 from arachidonic acid. PGH_2 is subsequently transformed to various isoforms, such as PGD_2, PGE_2, PGF_2 and PGI_2 (prostacyclin). In terms of pain and nociception, PGE_2 is the most extensively studied. Prostaglandins exert their effects by binding to specific receptors DP, EP, FP and IP for PGD_2, PGE_2, PGF_2 and PGI_2, respectively. All of them are G protein-coupled receptors (GPCR) that affect intracellular signaling by second messengers such as cAMP or inositol-triphosphate (IP_3). Four receptor subtypes for PGE_2 (EP1-EP4 receptors), with partially opposing signaling pathways, are responding to the naturally occurring agonist PGE_2 (Coleman et al., 1994).

Insofar PGE_2-induced central sensitization seems to be mediated by a COX-2-PGE_2 response to pro-inflammatory cytokines, resulting in phosphorylation and inhibition of the glycine receptor α3 in the superficial spinal cord dorsal horn (Vuilleumier et al., 2018).

This was recently confirmed in a murine model of inflammatory pain, where 2,6-Di-tert-buthylphenol reversed inflammation-mediated spinal nociception trough specific interaction with the phosphorylated glycine α 3 receptors, thereby reducing hyperalgesia (Acuña et al., 2016).

Spinal prostaglandins, particularly PGE_2, are involved in spinal nociception and sensitization. COX-1 and COX-2 are upregulated by painful stimuli, spinal PGE_2 causes pain and hyperalgesia, and these phenomena are attenuated by spinal application of COX-inhibitors or EP-antagonists. There is some evidence indicating similar effects in humans. Namely, Buvanendran and coauthors (2006) have investigated the relationship between postoperative pain in humans and prostaglandins in the cerebrospinal fluid. They demonstrated that IL-6 and PGE_2 increased markedly after total hip replacement. Moreover, the increase in PGE_2 was positively correlated to the intensity of postoperative pain, and preoperative administration of the COX-2 inhibitor *rofecoxib* was able to block this surgery-associated increase in PGE_2 (Buvanendran et al., 2006).

In conclusion, the central effects of NSAIDs are supported by a large body of evidence in animals. The central effects in inflammatory pain are robustly explained, whereby spinal inflammation-induced COX-2 expression and local PGE_2 concentration increases in the dorsal horn are linked to a decreased efficacy of inhibitory glycine-ergic interneurons that has recently confirmed by Vuilleumier et al., 2018. Neuropathic pain seems to be linked to mechanisms largely independent of the COX-2-PGE_2-EP2 pathway. Future research might address these questions using experimental settings other than spinal anesthesia with intrathecal NSAIDs. General anesthesia or measures of spinal hyper-excitability (e.g., nociceptive reflexes or temporal summation) might provide more insight. Translational research has nevertheless produced significant results since the first description of NSAID's spinal effects has increased our knowledge on the central prostaglandin E2 signaling pathway in inflammatory pain. Moreover, specific EP-antagonists might offer a novel approach to pain treatment, although their use is currently confined to the laboratory setting (Vuilleumier et al., 2018).

EMOTIONAL AWARENESS OF PAIN AND BRAIN LIMBIC AREAS

Functional neuroimaging investigations of pain have discovered a reliable pattern of activation within limbic regions of a putative "pain matrix" that has been theorized to reflect the emotional or affective dimension of pain. This pattern of activation includes regions of the PAG, thalamus, insula, ACC, amygdala and primary and secondary somatosensory cortices (SI/SII) (Feinstein et al., 2016; Morris et al., 2018). At the same time, the anterior, mid, and posterior division of the insula subserve different functions in the perception of pain. The anterior insula (AI) has predominantly been associated with cognitive–affective aspects of pain, while the mid and posterior divisions have been implicated in sensory-discriminative processing (Wiech et al., 2014).

To test this suggestion, it has been evaluated the experience of pain in a rare and unique neurological patient with extensive bilateral lesions encompassing core limbic structures of the pain matrix, including the insula, anterior cingulate, and amygdala. It was interesting and surprising that despite widespread damage to these regions, the patient's expression and experience of pain was intact, and at times excessive in nature. This finding was consistent across multiple pain measures including self-report, facial expression, vocalization, withdrawal reaction, and autonomic response. These results challenge the notion of a pain matrix and provide direct evidence that the insula, anterior cingulate, and amygdala are not necessary for feeling the suffering inherent to pain. The patient's heightened degree of pain affect further suggests that these regions may be more important for the regulation of pain rather than providing the decisive substrate for pain's conscious experience. In other words, the adaptive role of pain affect is so essential that the brain may automatically rewire in service of self-preservation. Consequently, the neural circuitry underlying pain and the associated feelings of suffering and distress is more complicated than previously thought, with multiple pathways and built-in redundancy allowing for maximal adaptation and resilience in the face of brain injury (Feinstein et al., 2016).

In the other study has been compared the analgesic effects of stimulation of the ACC or the posterior superior insula (PSI) against sham deep, repetitive transcranial magnetic stimulation (TMS) in ninety-eight patients with central neuropathic pain after stroke or spinal cord injury in a randomized, double-blinded, sham-controlled, 3-arm parallel study. They found that ACC- and PSI-deep TMS were not different from sham-deep TMS for pain relief in central neuropathic pain despite a significant antinociceptive effect after insular stimulation and anxiolytic effects of ACC-deep TMS. These results showed that the different dimensions of pain can be modulated in humans non-invasively by directly stimulating deeper *substantia nigra pars compacta* (SNC) structures without necessarily affecting clinical pain *per se* (Galhardoni et al., 2019).

Concerning the connectivity between insular subdivisions and other pain-related brain regions, functional neuroimaging studies have revealed that the AI division was predominantly connected to the ventro-lateral prefrontal cortex (structural and resting state connectivity) and orbito-frontal cortex (structural connectivity). In contrast, the posterior insula (PI) showed strong connections to the SI (structural connectivity) and SII (structural and resting state connectivity). The mid insula displayed a hybrid connectivity pattern with strong connections with the ventro-lateral prefrontal cortex, SII (structural and resting state connectivity) and SI (structural connectivity). Moreover, resting state connectivity revealed strong connectivity of all 3 subdivisions with the thalamus. On the behavioral level, AI structural connectivity was related to the individual degree of pain vigilance and awareness that showed a positive correlation with AI–amygdala connectivity and a negative correlation with AI–rACC connectivity. Overall, these findings showed a differential structural and resting state connectivity for the anterior, mid, and posterior insula with other pain-relevant brain regions, which might at least partly explain their different functional profiles in pain processing (Wiech et al., 2014).

Anatomical, behavioral and physiological evidences have indicated that the neuronal network in some key brain regions, including the ACC, prefrontal cortex (PFC), amygdala, bed nucleus stria terminalis and thalamus, processes information relating to the affective pain (Liu et al., 2018; Morris et al., 2018; Xiao, Zhang, 2018). For instance, connectivity between the ACC and subcortical structures including hypothalamic/preoptic nuclei and the bed nucleus of the stria terminalis correlated with the reduction in rats burrowing behavior observed following the persistent pain manipulation in a model of inflammatory arthritis pain (intra-articular injection of complete Freund's adjuvant) and measured ACC functional connectivity in the brain using fMRI. The findings therefore indicate a relatively specific relationship between ACC functional coupling and the suppression of burrowing behavior by persistent pain and suggest that ACC connectivity to these subcortical regions of the brain might be a good marker for the affective-motivational component of pain in rodents (Morris et al., 2018).

The dorsal part of the ACC is connected with the prefrontal cortex and parietal cortex as well as the motor system. By contrast, the ventral part of the ACC is connected with the AI, hypothalamus, amygdala, and nucleus accumbens. There is molecular link in between these related brain regions as well. The c-Fos expression associated with formalin-induced conditioned place avoidance (F-CPA) test occurred in the parabrachial nucleus (PBN), locus coeruleus (LC), PAG, amygdala, insular, prefrontal and anterior cingulate cortices (Xiao, Zhang, 2018). On the other hand, the BLA and the CeA are shown to play important roles in the integration of affective and sensory information including nociception. Using *in vivo* multichannel recording of neuronal discharges from the rACC and BLA, it has been shown that exposure of chronic forced swim stress to rats could result in an increased activity of rACC neuronal population and promote the functional connectivity and the synchronization between rACC and BLA regions, and also enhance the pain–related neural information flow from rACC to BLA, which likely underlie the pathogenesis of stress-induced hyperalgesia (Liu et al., 2018).

The antinociceptive effects of the endogenous fatty acid amide, N-palmitoylethanolamide (PEA), in the peripheral and CNSs have been demonstrated in numerous studies employing animal models of inflammatory and neuropathic pain (Guida et al., 2015; Okine et al., 2014). It has recently found in rats that intra-ACC administration of PEA significantly attenuated the first and early second phases of formalin-evoked nociceptive behavior. This effect was attenuated by the CB1 receptor antagonist AM-251, but not by the peroxisome proliferator-activated receptor (PPAR) isoform alpha (PPARα) antagonist GW6471, the PPARγ antagonist GW9662, or the TRPV1 (transient receptor potential vanilloid 1) channel antagonist 5′-iodo resiniferatoxin (a potent functional analog of capsaicin). All antagonists administered alone, significantly reduced formalin-evoked nociceptive behavior, suggesting facilitatory/permissive roles for these receptors in the ACC in inflammatory pain. Post-mortem tissue analysis revealed a strong trend for increased levels of the endocannabinoid anandamide (AEA) in the ACC of rats that received intra-ACC PEA. Expression of c-Fos, a marker of neuronal activity, was significantly reduced in the basolateral nucleus of the amygdala (BLA), but not in the CeA, the rostral ventromedial medulla (RVM) or the dorsal horn of the spinal cord. These data indicated that PEA in the ACC can reduce inflammatory pain-related behavior, possibly *via* AEA-induced activation of CB1 receptors and associated modulation of neuronal activity in the basolateral amygdala (Okine et al., 2016).

The role of PPAR signaling in the development or modulation of human chronic pain conditions, such as cancer pain, osteoarthritis, diabetic neuropathy, and migraine requires further study, as does the interaction of PPAR signaling with other well characterized endogenous pain control systems and currently prescribed analgesics. On this latter point, the PPARγ agonist *pioglitazone* has been shown to attenuate tolerance to morphine in a rat model of inflammatory pain and in the mouse tail immersion test. Similar potential synergistic antinociceptive interactions with the cannabinoid and TRPV1 channel signaling systems have been reported. In respect of the latter study, the evidence suggests that the potential antinociceptive effects of this synergistic interaction are likely to be facilitated by PPARα-dependent activation of TRPV1 channels and subsequent desensitization of the receptor. Elsewhere, a synergistic antinociceptive interaction between PEA and the opiate drug, *tramadol*, has been demonstrated in the mouse formalin test. The antinociceptive mechanisms of the PEA and tramadol combination involved the opioid receptor, TRPV1 and PPARα. Significantly, the sedative effects of the combination of PEA and tramadol were minimal compared with those observed with individual treatments. Collectively, these findings make a compelling case for an increased understanding of PPAR signaling and its crosstalk with other analgesic targets. Such knowledge could lead to the development of novel PPAR signaling based-analgesic strategies" (Okine et al., 2019).

BRAIN LIMBIC AREAS IN PAIN CHRONIFICATION

Pain pathways represent a complex sensory system with cognitive, emotional, and behavioral influences. Anatomically, the hippocampus, amygdala, and anterior cortex including cingulate cortex, – central to the encoding and consolidation of memory, – are also implicated in experiential aspects of pain. Common neurotransmitters and similar mechanisms of neural plasticity (e.g., central sensitization, long-term potentiation) suggest a mechanistic overlap between chronic pain and memory. These anatomic and mechanistic correlates indicate that chronic pain and memory intimately interact on several levels. Longitudinal imaging studies suggest that spatiotemporal reorganization of brain activity accompanies the transition to chronic pain, during which the representation of pain gradually shifts from sensory to emotional and limbic structures (McCarberg, Peppin, 2019). The interaction of limbic–cortical circuits identified by neuro-imaging studies is consistent with the concept of close interaction between pain, memory, and learning. In this regard, we can consider pain as memory or one of the varieties of memory (Tsagareli, 2013).

Pain receptors (nociceptors) signal input to the spinal cord and supraspinal structures, triggering a prolonged but reversible increase in the excitability and synaptic efficacy of neurons in central nociceptive pathways, is the phenomenon of central sensitization. Key processes for pain memory stabilizing could be considering processes of peripheral and central sensitizations. During peripheral and central sensitization, the receptive fields of dorsal horn neurons expand beyond the site of injury into surrounding non-injured tissue. The clinical result of all the above changes is hyperalgesia, allodynia, spontaneous pain, referred pain, and sympathetically maintained pain. Therefore, these persistent sensory responses to noxious stimuli are a form of memory, the memory for pain. Long- lasting synaptic plasticity as the long-term potentiation at spinal and supraspinal levels could undergo hyperalgesia and allodynia. The latter could be providing the neuronal basis for persistent pain and pain memory. Thus, it will be particularly important to know mechanisms of long-lasting plastic changes in the spinal cord, thalamus, and cortex. The molecular machinery of these plastic processes could be main targets for new therapeutic drugs in pain relief (Tsagareli, 2013).

In the model proposed by research group of Apkarian (Mansour et al., 2014), chronic pain is suffering that fails to extinguish its memory trace, and instead reflects a state of continuous learning in which the interaction between the prefrontal cortex and limbic learning circuitry is central to the transition to chronicity (Figure 35). In this model transient nociceptive signals mainly evoke acute pain perception through activation of the anterior cingulate cortex and insular cortex and limbic–cortical plasticity underlies the shift to chronic pain. They suggested that normally any learned associations mediated by the limbic circuitry would be gradually extinguished or unlearned with time. However, the limbic circuitry could be preferentially activated (including the amygdala, hippocampus, and nucleus accumbens) if the nociceptive signal was persistent and/or intense. These structures are integral to learning and memory. In turn, these pathways shift cortical activity from a predominately nociceptive state to a more emotional one by interacting with the prefrontal cortical circuitry, with pain transitioning to a more emotional state. The limbic circuitry also provides modulatory signals to the cortex, causing functional and anatomical alterations (Figure 35) (Mansour et al., 2014). According to this hypothesis, the persistence of pain-related perceptions is driven by implicit and explicit memories interacting with subconscious signals. Thereby, chronic pain is either "unlearned" or maintained depending on the reaction of the mesolimbic emotional learning circuitry. The limbic–cortical circuitry impacts descending modulatory pathways thereby influencing spinal cord responses to nociceptive inputs. Thus, the process of chronification of pain involves interactions at multiple levels of CNS and offers several possible therapeutic targets. Increased understanding of the neurophysiology of chronic pain has provided insight into potential prophylactic and treatment strategies that prevent the establishment of chronic pain pathways or reverse the reorganization that accompanies chronic pain including regions involved in memory and learning (McCarberg, Peppin, 2019).

Brain structures, including the primary and secondary somatosensory cortices (SI/SII), prefrontal cortex (PFC), anterior cingulate cortex (ACC), insular cortex (IC), amygdala, thalamus, and of periaqueductal grey matter (PAG) and rostral ventro-medial medulla (RVM), have been identified as regions associated with the perception of pain. The ventral tegmental area (VTA) and nucleus accumbens (NAc), structures comprising the mesolimbic reward circuit, are involved in chronic pain. The prefrontal region and limbic system (ACC, amygdala, VTA, and NAc) are also associated with affective aspects of pain and regulate emotional and motivational responses (Figure 35) (Mansour et al., 2014). These brain regions are not activated separately but are functionally connected and contribute in a combined fashion to pain processing. Changes in emotional and motivational cues can affect the intensity and degree of pain experience (Apkarian et al., 2005; Bushnell et al., 2013; Leknes, Tracey, 2008; Navratilova et al., 2016; Yang, Chang, 2019).

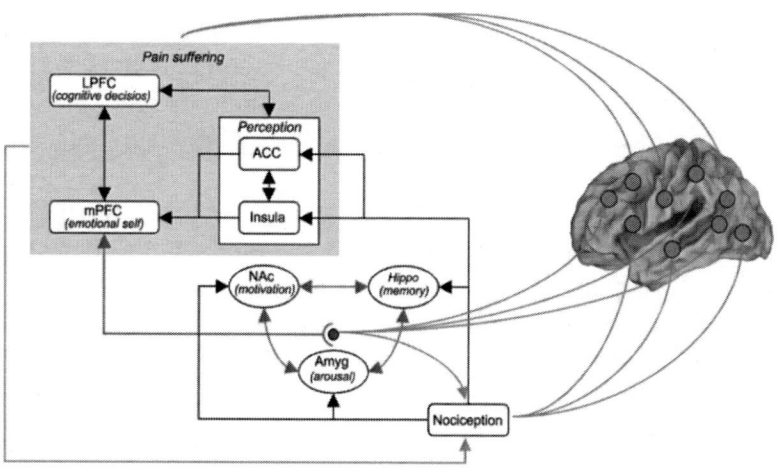

Figure 35. A model of the brain circuitry involved in the transition from acute to chronic pain. Schematic connections between pain key structures correspond to the points in the brain illustration. Abbreviations: ACC, anterior cingulate cortex; Amyg, amygdala; Hippo, hippocampus; lPFC, lateral prefrontal cortex; mPFC, medial prefrontal cortex; NAc, nucleus accumbens. (Reproduced from Mansour et al., 2014, with permission).

To date, several studies have demonstrated the high comorbidity of affective disorders in patients with chronic pain. Many patients with chronic pain also have severe depression. Patients with chronic pain-induced depression have poorer prognosis than those with chronic pain alone (Yang, Chang, 2019). Chronic pain and depression share similar changes in neuroplasticity and involve overlapping neurobiological mechanisms; monoamine neurotransmitters such as serotonin, dopamine, and norepinephrine are decreased in both chronic pain and depression patients. Additionally, brain regions involved in pain pathways, such as the PFC, hippocampus, and amygdala, are similar to those involved in mood disorders (Bair et al., 2003; Haase, Brown, 2018; Sheng et al., 2017).

As pain develops into a chronic condition, negative emotional states may be accompanied by other emotional disorders such as anxiety, anhedonia, cognitive deficits, sleep disturbances, and suicide (Apkarian et al., 2005; Elman et al., 2013). The prevalence of suicidal ideation and suicide attempts is noticeably higher in patients with chronic pain than in control patients (Fishbain et al., 2014). A recent review indicated that chronic pain itself is an important independent risk factor for suicidality regardless of type and concluded that depressive symptoms, anger problems, and harmful habits are general risk factors for suicidality in patients with chronic pain (Racine, 2018).

Several animal studies have also demonstrated the negative affective disorders associated with pain. A study using a rat model with a chronic constriction injury (CCI) reported that long-term pain led to an anxiety-like profile, increased responses to aversion, and impairments in cognitive tasks (Llorca-Torralba et al., 2019; Yang, Chang, 2019). It has recently reported that negative affects including pain aversion and anxiety were associated with hyperalgesia but that the manifestations of negative effects may occur over different time courses, suggesting that therapy should be targeted based on the different stages of pain and its comorbidities (Wu et al., 2017). Chronic pain and various affective disorders are often managed poorly, therefore, understanding the affective aspects related to chronic pain may facilitate the development of novel therapies for more effective management (Yang, Chang, 2019).

Pain chronification, thus, is accompanied by spatio-temporal reorganization of brain activity, with a transition from sensory regions to emotional and motivational areas of the limbic brain (McCarberg, Peppin, 2019). As we stated here, the cortico-limbic system is a mediator of chronic pain and plays an important role in the development, maintenance, and amplification of chronic pain (Apkarian et al., 2009; Vachon-Presseau et al., 2016). Structural and functional plasticity in the cortico-limbic circuitry accompanies the transition from acute to chronic pain. When nociceptive signals persist, the cortico-limbic circuitry stays activated. Through the interactions with the prefrontal cortical circuitry, nociceptive state progresses to a more emotional state. The persistent activation of the cortico-limbic circuitry brings functional and anatomic alterations to the cortex, resulting in pain chronification (Mansour et al., 2014; Yang, Chang, 2019).

The medial PFC is an important region for top-down cognitive control over emotion-driven behaviors and is a critical region involved in emotional and cognitive processing in chronic pain (Kang et al., 2019; Thompson, Neugebauer, 2019). The prelimbic and infralimbic medial PFCs receive inputs from brain regions, including the basolateral amygdala (BLA), hippocampus, thalamus, and contralateral medial PFC, send excitatory projections to the amygdala (Thompson, Neugebauer, 2019). Chronic pain is considered to develop as a result of the persistence of pain memory and inability to erase pain memory after injury (Apkarian et al., 2009). Considering its importance in extinction of fear behaviors, impaired medial PFC activation could lead to a failure in the elimination of subcortically driven fear behaviors, thereby resulting in pain chronification (Thompson, Neugebauer, 2019; Yang, Chang, 2019).

The amygdala associated with emotions and affective disorders, plays an important role in emotional affective aspects of pain (Kato et al., 2018; Neugebauer, 2015; Simons et al., 2014; Thompson, Neugebauer, 2017; Vachon-Presseau et al., 2016). The amygdala receives cortical and thalamic inputs, and the lateral/basolateral (LA/BLA) complex of the amygdala adds emotional and affective context to sensory information. This information is then sent to the CeA, which comprises GABA-ergic neurons and regulates fear and pain (Neugebauer, 2015; Thompson, Neugebauer, 2017, 2019; Yang, Chang, 2019).

It is well known that the hippocampus as part of the limbic system plays an important role in declarative and episodic memory (Aggleton, Morris, 2018; Eichenbaum, 2017). On the other hand, changes in the hippocampus have been reported in chronic pain conditions. In particular, hippocampal neurogenesis contributes to learning and memory and may trigger the development of chronic pain. The upregulation of hippocampal neurogenesis resulted in the prolongation of persistent pain (Apkarian et al., 2016). In addition, chronic pain is generally accompanied by cognitive deficits and aversive emotional states, including depression and anxiety disorders. Functional and structural changes in the hippocampus, such as decreased hippocampal neurogenesis, are closely associated with memory deficits and aversive affective states in patients with chronic pain (Apkarian et al., 2016; Thompson, Neugebauer, 2019; Yang, Chang, 2019).

The ACC is also associated with affective and motivational aspects of pain, and involved in the processing and modulation of pain (Navratilova et al., 2015; Neugebauer, 2015). Nociceptive inputs are sent from the medial thalamus to ACC and combined with motivation and affective information received from other brain areas, such as the IC, medial PFC, and BLA (Baliki, Apkarian, 2015; Bushnell et al., 2013; Navratilova et al., 2015; Thompson, Neugebauer, 2019). The ACC then generates affective and motivational pain responses through its projections to the amygdala, NAc, and medial PFC. Additionally, the interactions of the ACC with pain neuro-circuitry in the PAG have been reported, which accounts for the activation of the ACC and PAG in the presence of noxious stimuli. The activation of ACC-PFC-PAG circuity and increased activity in the ACC is associated with negative emotions (Baliki, Apkarian, 2015; Bushnell et al., 2013; Navratilova et al., 2015; Thompson, Neugebauer, 2019; Yang, Chang, 2019).

In the second chapter we emphasized that the midcingulate division of the cingulate cortex (MCC) does not mediate acute pain sensation and pain affect, but gates sensory hypersensitivity by acting in a wide cortical and subcortical network (Tan et al., 2017). Within this complex network, an afferent MCC–PI (posterior insula) pathway that can induce and maintain nociceptive hypersensitivity in the absence of conditioned peripheral noxious drive. This facilitation of nociception is brought about by recruitment of descending serotoninergic facilitatory projections to the spinal cord. The PI is anatomically and functionally connected with the raphe magnus nucleus, the site of origin of serotoninergic modulation, and found that the MCC–PI pathway influenced nociception by recruiting descending serotoninergic mechanisms. Serotoninergic pathways originating in the nucleus raphe magnus (NRM) exert prominent facilitatory modulation in the spinal cord (Tan et al., 2017). These results have implications for understanding of neuronal mechanisms facilitating the transition from acute to persistent, long-lasting pain (Figure 4) (Nevian, 2017).

The key structure of pain modulation is the PAG located in the brain stem. It is divided into three subregions: ventrolateral, lateral, and dorsolateral, and plays an important role in both the ascending and descending modulation of nociception, and of regulates other autonomic and emotional behaviors. It connects to the rostral ventromedial medulla (RVM), which sends descending inhibitory and excitatory fibers to the dorsal horn of the spinal cord. The PAG integrates information received from higher centers of the brain and receives ascending nociceptive input from the dorsal horn (Figure 36) (Chen, Heinricher, 2019). The PAG regulates the processing of nociceptive information in the dorsal horn of the spinal cord and plays a critical role in the descending modulation of pain (Hemington, Coulombe, 2015; Holstege, 2014; Yang, Chang, 2019).

Finally, the PAG proposing to function as the gateway for pain control from higher brain centers to the spinal cord, does not project directly to the spinal cord and uses a relay located at the RVM. The RVM exerts dual actions, i.e., inhibitory and facilitatory, leading to balance of inhibition (antinociception) and facilitation (pronociception) of noxious signal transmission at the spinal cord. The imbalance between inhibition and facilitation towards the spinal cord accounts for chronic pain installation. The NRM is a structure in the RVM that is a major site in the endogenous pain inhibitory system that receives projections from the PAG. The NRM comprises one of the main serotoninergic neuronal populations in the brain and is the principal source of fibers containing serotonin at the spinal cord. The depletion of serotoninergic neurons in the NRM was shown to reduce nociceptive behaviors in animal models of traumatic neuropathic pain (Costa-Pereira et al., 2020).

Different types neurotransmitters (inflammatory mediators, including prostaglandin E2, adenosine triphosphate, adenosine, histamine, glutamate, and nitric oxide (NO), or non-inflammatory mediators, including GABA, CGRP, peptides, glycine, and cannabinoids) are involved in pain transmission in either an inhibitory or excitatory way. Nervous and glial cells, such as microglia and astrocytes, release various neurotransmitters that contribute to the development and maintenance of chronic pain by activating or deactivating nociceptive neurons in the CNS (Carniglia et al., 2017; Ji et al., 2013; Yam et al., 2018).

General Discussion

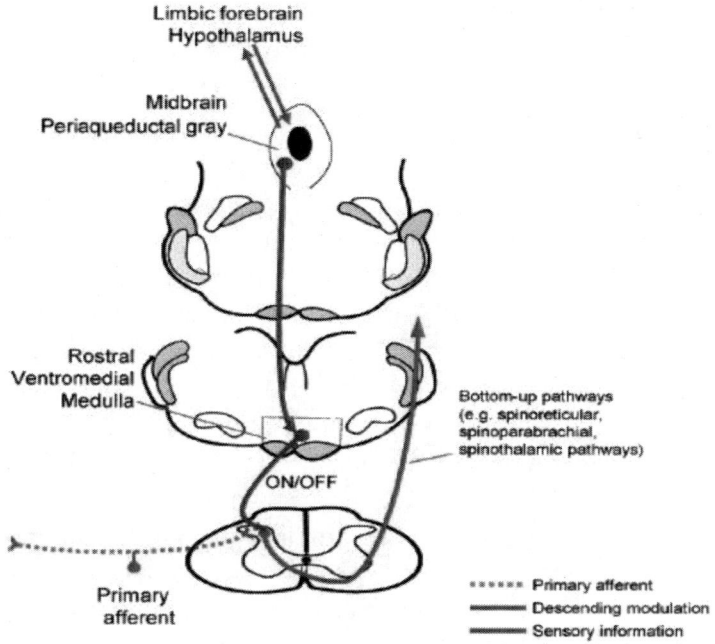

Figure 36. The PAG-RVM descending pain-modulating pathway exerts facilitatory and inhibitory drive on dorsal horn neurons. The output of this pathway can be influenced by higher structures, such as hypothalamus and limbic forebrain. (Reproduced from Chen, Heinricher, 2019, with permission).

A wide range of neuropeptides (neuropeptide Y, vasoactive intestinal peptide (VIP), cortistatin, somatostatin, tachykinins, CGRP, ghrelin and adrenomedullin) play various roles in the formation, transmission, modulation, and perception of different types of pain. These neuropeptides bind to specific receptors expressed on microglial cells and influence pain processes, including neuro-inflammation, neurodegeneration, and neuro-modulation (Yang, Chang, 2019).

Opioid peptides are a family of neuropeptides that bind to opioid receptors, including mu, delta and kappa receptor subtypes (Azzam et al., 2019). Opioid receptors are abundantly distributed in both primary afferent neurons and dendrites of postsynaptic neurons. Enkephalin and dynorphin are two endogenous opioid peptides that inhibit the release of excitatory neurotransmitters from afferent terminals and reduce neuronal excitability, resulting in decreased pain sensation (Yam et al., 2018). Changes in the capacity of brain regions to respond to endogenous or exogenous opioids are related to decrease opioid receptor expression, which may underscore the lack of efficacy of opioids in chronic pain. Reduced opioid receptor availability, reflecting decreased receptor expression, contributes to the development of chronic pain (Brown et al., 2015).

Endocannabinoids are a class of neurotransmitters present in pain signal transduction pathways and regulate neural conduction of pain signals by attenuating sensitization and inflammation *via* the activation of cannabinoid CB1 and CB2 receptors, which are located at peripheral, spinal, or supraspinal sites (Piomelli, Sasso, 2014). Cannabinoid receptors modulate neuro-immune interactions and inflammatory hyperalgesia when endo- or exogenous-cannabinoids inhibit the release of presynaptic neurotransmitters and neuropeptides, modulate postsynaptic neuronal excitability, activate descending inhibitory pathways, and reduce neuro-inflammatory signaling (Hill et al., 2017; Jimenez, 2018; Starowicz, Finn, 2017). Long-term studies evaluating treatment effects of exogenous cannabinoids should take into consideration the efficacy, therapeutic window, dose-dependent effects, and side effects to provide support for the use of cannabinoids in pain treatment (Jimenez, 2018).

In conclusion, in order to develop appropriate therapeutic targets for chronic pain, it is important to understand factors that affect the transition of acute pain to chronic pain and the mechanisms underlying the development of chronic pain. The development of chronic pain is associated with sensitization and synaptic plasticity in various brain areas such as the PFC, ACC, IC, amygdala, hippocampus, NAc, and PAG. In the future, should investigate factors that trigger pain chronification to provide insight into how acute pain becomes chronic. Therefore, a deeper understanding of the mechanisms and key factors involved in pain chronification is necessary to identify novel therapeutic targets for developing better treatments for chronic pain avoiding side effects like tolerance (Yang, Chang, 2019).

Chapter 9

SUMMARY AND CONCLUSION

The limbic system firstly described by Papez (1937) and then expanded by MacLean (1952), is a complex set of structures that lies on both sides of the thalamus, just under the cerebrum. It includes the hypothalamus, hippocampus, amygdala, insula, cingulum and several others nearby areas. It appears to be primarily responsible for emotional life, and has a lot to do with the formation of memories. The limbic system produces the emotions that can often accompany pain, such as anxiety or fear, often affecting the way the cerebral cortex receives pain messages and lessening or intensifying the pain feeling.

The wealth of imaging studies (Bushnell et al., 2013; Casey, 2000; Kuner, Flor, 2017; Leknes, Tracey 2008; Xu et al., 2020) showing alterations in the brain limbic areas of patients with chronic pain can now be integrated with increased understanding of the brain circuitry involved in the psychological modulation of pain, allowing to hypothesize a negative-feedback loop between impaired pain modulatory circuitry and pain processing, leading not only to increased chronic pain but also to cognitive and emotional deficits that are comorbid with the pain (Bushnell et al., 2013).

Concerning the pain relief, cannabinoids and opioids produce antinociceptive synergy. Cannabinoids such as delta-9-tetrahydro-cannabinol (THC) release endogenous opioids and endocannabinoids such as anandamide (N-arachidonoylethanolamine, AEA) also alter endogenous opioid analgesia. Opioids and cannabinoids bind distinct receptors that co-localize in areas of the brain involved in the processing of pain signals (Welch, 2009). Therefore, it is logical to look at interactions of these two systems in the modulation of both acute and chronic pain. These drugs are often co-abused. In addition, the lack of continued effectiveness of opioids due to tolerance development limits the use of such drugs. The data indicate that with cannabinoid/opioid therapy one may be able to produce long-term antinociceptive effects at doses devoid of substantial side effects, while preventing the neuronal biochemical changes that accompany tolerance. The clinical utility of modulators of the endocannabinoid system as a potential mimic for THC-like drugs in analgesia and tolerance-sparing effects of opioids is a critical future direction, i.e., effective antinociception with delayed development tolerance (Desroches, Beaulieu, 2010; Desroches et al., 2014; Nielsen et al., 2017; Welch, 2009).

In this book, we presented new data indicating that microinjections of widely used non-opioid, NSAID analgesics diclofenac, ketoprofen, ketorolac, and lornoxicam into pain matrix key structures of brain limbic areas, such as the rostral part of the anterior cingulate cortex, agranular insular cortex, and central nucleus of amygdala of rats induced antinociception. When administered repeatedly, tolerance developed to the antinociceptive effects of these drugs. Pre- or post-treatment with opioid receptor antagonists, naloxone and CTOP as well as cannabinoid CB1 receptor antagonist AM-251, separately or in combination in the CeA, prevented or abolished antinociceptive effects of these non-opioid analgesics. On the basis of our findings, we confirmed the concept that antinociception and the development of tolerance to NSAIDs are mediated *via* endogenous opioid and cannabinoid systems involving the descending pain modulatory circuits attenuating pain behavior in rats – defensive withdrawal reflexes at the spinal cord level. The crucial structures of this descending pain modulatory system are midbrain periaqueductal grey matter (PAG) and rostral ventromedial medulla (RVM).

In particular, the ventro-lateral column of the PAG forms part of a descending analgesic pathway that projects *via* the RVM to the spinal dorsal horn where it inhibits ascending nociceptive transmission to the brain. According to last findings, mu-opioids activate the descending analgesic pathway from the midbrain PAG by a combination of presynaptic disinhibition of RVM-projecting neurons and postsynaptic inhibition of presumptive interneurons. Thus, the opioid disinhibition is pleiotropic, involving both postsynaptic inhibition of intrinsic PAG neurons and presynaptic inhibition of their outputs onto descending projection neurons in the RVM. In this regard, presynaptic and postsynaptic opioid receptors couple *via* different intracellular pathways and effectors. This is likely to have implications for the chronic use of opioids for pain management because presynaptic opioid receptors display different levels and mechanisms of desensitization compared to postsynaptic receptors. In this way, a better understanding of the interactions between presynaptic and postsynaptic opioid signaling in brain antinociceptive systems is required to improve opioid analgesic drugs (Lau et al., 2020).

It was well known that the analgesic effects of non-opioid, NSAIDs are due to their action on three major sites, namely, peripheral inflamed tissues, spinal cord, and the brain stem. However, our study clearly showed that NSAIDs exerted on the brain limbic areas as well, producing robust antinociception, and in repeated microinjections antinociceptive tolerance. These data, thus, emphasized the important role of these limbic regions, the rostral anterior cingulate cortex, agranular insular cortex, and central amygdala in rats' pain behavior.

Chapter 10

METHODOLOGY
(MATERIALS AND METHODS)

ANIMALS

The research was carried out on adult male Wistar rats weighing 200–250 g, bred at the Beritashvili Center for Experimental Biomedicine (BMC). The animals were kept under standard housing conditions (22°C ± 2°C, 65% humidity, light from 7:00 a.m. to 8:00p.m.), and kept on a standard dry diet with water freely available. Every effort was made to minimize both the number of animals used and their suffering. Six rats were used for each experimental and control group. The local Bioethic Committee of the BMC approved the experimental protocols, and we adhered to the Guidelines of the International Association for the Study of Pain (IASP) regarding investigations of experimental pain in conscious animals (Zimmermann, 1983).

SURGICAL PROCEDURES

Under anesthesia with intramuscular administration of ketamine (100 mg/kg, "KharkovPharm," Ukraine), a 12-mm-long stainless steel guide cannula (Small Parts, Inc., Logansport, IN, USA) was stereotaxically implanted bilaterally into the rostral part of AIC, (AP: 2.70; L: ±4.4; H: 5.8), the CeA (AP: –1.8; L: +8; H: 3.8), and of monolaterally into the rostral part of ACC (area I) (AP: 2.70; L: +0.5; H: 2.5), according to the coordinates in the atlas of Paxinos and Watson (1997), siting the tip 2 mm above a given structure. The guides were anchored to the cranium using dental cement. The guide cannula was plugged with a stainless-steel stylet. Thereafter, the animals were handled every day for 3–4 days for 15–20 minutes to get familiar with the testing protocol and experimental environment. During this time, the stylet was removed and a 14-mm long stainless-steel microinjection cannula was inserted into the guide cannula to reach the AIC, but no drug was injected. Five days after surgery, the microinjection cannula, attached to Hamilton syringe (Hamilton, Inc., McLean, VA, USA), was joined to the guide cannula, and the drug was introduced through it while the rat was gently restrained.

DRUGS

Diclofenac (clodifen, diclofenac sodium, 75 μg/0.5 μL, Hemofarm, Vršac, Serbia), ketorolac (ketorolac tromethamine, 90 μg/0.5 μL, Grindex, Latvia), ketoprofen (ketonal, 25 μg/0.5 μl, Sandoz, Slovenia), or lornoxicam (xefocam, 12 μg/0.5 μL, Nycomed, Zürich, Austria) were injected through the microinjection cannula as used in previous works (Pirkulashvili et al., 2017; Tsiklauri et al., 2018a, b). The guide cannula was then plugged with a stainless-steel stylet. Isotonic saline was injected in the same volume (0.5 μL, GalichPharm, Ukraine) and manner in a separate group of rats, treated as controls. In the second set of experiments, a nonselective opioid receptor antagonist naloxone (0.2 μg/0.5 μL, Polfa S.A., Poland), a selective mu-opioid receptor antagonist CTOP (octapeptide, D-Phe-Cys-Tyr-D-Trp-Orn-Thr-Pen-Thr-$_{NH2}$) (100 ng/0.5 μl, Sigma-Aldrich), and of the cannabinoid 1 (CB1) receptor antagonist AM-251 (1 μM/0.5 μl, Sigma-Aldrich, St. Louis, MO, USA) were injected through the microinjection cannula. Solutions were microinjected in about 10–15 seconds.

Methodology (Materials and Methods)

BEHAVIORAL TESTING

Twenty minutes after microinjection of NSAIDs or saline, i.e., 10 minutes before the peak of the drugs' effect is normally reached, rats were tested for antinociception using rodent's behavior tests for assessment the effects of drugs in the acute or smooth pain models, among them the 'formalin test.'

- *Tail-flick test (TF).* For the TF test, the distal part of the tail was stimulated with a light beam and the latency measured until the tail was reflexively flicked away from the beam (IITC #33, IITC Life Science, Inc., Woodland Hills, CA, USA).
- *Hot plate test (HP).* For the HP test, the rat was placed on a 55°C hot plate and the latency to the first hindpaw lick or time to first jump was measured (IITC #39). The cut off time was 20 s for both TF and HP latencies. Each rat was tested for both TF and HP latencies in the same session. A similar procedure was followed for the repeated microinjection of NSAIDs or saline for four or five consecutive days.
- *Thermal paw withdrawal (Hargreaves) test.* For Hargreaves' test (IITC #390, IITC Life science, Inc., Woodland Hills, CA, USA) rats were first habituated over three successive daily sessions to stand on a glass surface heated to 30 ± 1 °C within a ventilated Plexiglas enclosure. Before formal testing, baseline latencies for paw withdrawals evoked by radiant thermal stimulation were measured five times per paw, with at least 5 min intervals between tests of a given paw. A light beam was focused onto the plantar surface of the hindpaw through a glass plate from below, and the latency from onset of the light to brisk withdrawal of the stimulated paw was measured. To prevent potential tissue damage, a cutoff time of 20 s was used if no paw movement occurred.
- *Mechanical paw withdrawal threshold (von Frey) test.* For von Frey test (IITC Life science, Inc., USA) baseline mechanical withdrawal thresholds were assessed using an electronic von Frey filament with 90 g range (#1601C, IITC) pressed against the plantar surface of one hindpaw. This device registered the force

(g) at the moment that the hindpaw was withdrawn from the filament.

In different studies, each animal was tested with both TF and HP tests in the same session, and with Hargreaves and von Frey tests in different sessions. Similar procedures were followed for the repeated microinjection of diclofenac (clodifen), ketorolac, ketoprofen (ketonal) and lornoxicam (xefocam), or saline for four consecutive days.

In the second set of experiments, pretreatment of rats with naloxone, CTOP or AM-251 in the above-mentioned brain limbic structures (rACC, AIC, or CeA) was followed by TF and HP, or Hargreaves and von Frey tests. 10-15 minutes after they were treated with NSAIDs in the same dose as in the first set of experiments and were then retested again.

In the third set of experiments, post-treatment of rats with naloxone, CTOP, or AM-251 in the AIC, rACC or CeA were followed by TF and HP, or Hargreaves and von Frey tests. For this purpose, 10-15 minutes prior to opioid receptors antagonist or CB1 receptor antagonist were microinjected, rats were pretreated with NSAIDs in the same dose as in the first and second set of experiments and were then retested again. Different animal groups were used for the first, second, and third sets of experiments. The number of rats in each group was six.

- *Formalin-induced nociception test.* Rats were placed in plastic cylinders on a room temperature glass surface and allowed to acclimate for approximately one hour before injection. The formalin solution was prepared at 10% in saline from a formalin stock (Sigma-Aldrich, USA) and a unilateral intraplantar injection (right hindpaw) was made in a volume of 50 ml. The formalin stock corresponded to a 37% formaldehyde solution. In rodents, intraplantar injections of formalin produce a biphasic behavioral reaction consisting of an initial phase of paw-flinching occurring about 3–5 min after the injection the acute pain), followed by a quiescent period, a then second phase of flinching beginning after 20–30 min (the smooth pain). The intensities of these behaviors are dependent on the concentration of formalin that is administered. We presently collected data at minute 5 post-formalin injections representing the first phase, and at minutes

15 and 45 post-NSAIDs injections, i.e., at minutes 30 and 60 post-formalin injections representing the second phase.

HISTOLOGY

At the end of each set of experiments, the microinjection sites were marked with 2 μl of saturated solution of Direct Blue-1 (Sigma-Aldrich) and the animal was euthanized with pentobarbital. After fixation by immersion in 10% formalin, the brain was sectioned and counterstained with Cresyl Violet. The microinjection sites were histologically verified and plotted according to Paxinos and Watson (1997) stereotaxic atlas coordinates.

STATISTICAL ANALYSIS

All data are presented as mean ± S.E.M. One-way analysis of variance (ANOVA) or repeated measures of ANOVA (rMANOVA) with post-hoc Tukey-Kramer or Dannett's multiple comparison tests were used for statistical comparisons between NSAIDs treated and saline groups, and NSAIDs treated and opioid and cannabinoid (CB1) receptors antagonists (naloxone, CTOP or AM-251) groups, respectively. For a comparison selected pairs of columns we used Bonferroni Multiple Comparison Test. The Kolmogorov–Smirnov test was applied to verify normality. For some group differences we also used unpaired two-tailed t-tests. The statistical software utilized was InStat 3.05 (GraphPad Software, USA). Differences between means of vehicle control and all NSAIDs treated groups or between NSAIDs and antagonist treated groups of rats were acknowledged as statistically significant if $P < 0.05$.

REFERENCES

Abrams D. I., Guzman M. (2015) Cannabis in cancer care. *Clin Pharmacol Therap,* 97(6): 575-586 (doi: 10.1002/cpt.108).

Abrams D. I., Couey P., Shade S. B., Kelly M. E., Benowitz N. L. (2011) Cannabinoid–opioid interaction inchronic pain. *Clin Pharmacol Ther,* 90 (6): 844-851 (doi: 10.1038/clpt.2011.188).

Acuña M. A., Yévenes G. E., Ralvenius W. T., Benke D., Di Lio A., Lara C. O. et al. (2016) Phosphorylation state-dependent modulation of spinal glycine receptors alleviates inflammatory pain. *J Clin Invest,* 126(7): 2547– 2560 (doi: 10.1172/JCI83817).

Aggleton J. P., Morris R. G. M. (2018) Memory: Looking back and looking forward. *Brain Neurosci Adv,* 2: 1-9 (doi: 10.1177/2398212818794483).

Al Amin H. A., Atweh S. F., Jabbur S. J., Saade N. E. (2004) Effects of ventral hippocampal lesion on thermal and mechanical nociception in neonates and adult rats. *Eur J Neurosci,* 20(11): 3027–3034 (doi: 10.1111/j.1460-9568.2004.03762.x).

Alter B. J., Gereau R. W. (2008) Hotheaded: TRPV1 as mediator of hippocampal synaptic plasticity. *Neuron,* 57(5): 629-631 (doi: 10.1016/j.neuron.2008.02.023).

Amanzio M, Palermo S. (2019) Pain anticipation and nocebo-related responses: A descriptive mini-review of functional neuroimaging studies in normal subjects and precious hints on pain processing in the context of neurodegenerative disorders. *Front Pharmacol,* 10: 969 (doi: 10.3389/fphar.2019.00969).

Apkarian A. V. (2019) Definitions of nociception, pain, and chronic pain with implications regarding science and society. *Neurosci Letters,* 702: 1-2 (doi: 10.1016/j.neulet.2018.11.039).

Apkarian A. V., Baliki M. N., Geha P. Y. (2009) Towards a theory of chronic pain. *Prog Neurobiol,* 87(2): 81–97 (doi: 10.1016/j.pneurobio.2008.09.018).

Apkarian A. V., Bushnell M. C., Treede R. D., Zubieta J. K. (2005) Human brain mechanisms of pain perception and regulation in health and disease. *Eur J Pain,* 9(4): 463–484 (doi: 10.1016/j.ejpain.2004.11.001).

Apkarian A. V., Mutso A. A., Centeno, M. V., Kan L., Wu M., Levinstein M. et al. (2016) Role of adult hippocampal neurogenesis in persistent pain. *Pain,* 157(2): 418–428 (doi: 10.1097/j.pain.0000000000000332).

Araque A., Castillo P.E., Manzoni O.J., Tonini R. (2017) Synaptic functions of endocannabinoid signaling in health and disease. *Neuropharmacol,* 124: 13-24 (doi: 10.1016/j.neuropharm.2017.06.017).

Azzam A. A. H., McDonald J., Lambert D. G. (2019) Hot topics in opioid pharmacology: Mixed and biased opioids. *Brit J Anaesthesiol,* 122(6): e136–e145 (doi: 10.1016/j.bja.2019.03.006).

Bair M. J., Robinson R. L., Katon W., Kroenke K. (2003) Depression and pain comorbidity: A literature review. *Arch Intern Med,* 163(20): 2433–2445 (doi: 10.1001/archinte.163.20.2433).

Ballantyne J. C., Sullivan M. D. (2017) Discovery of endogenous opioid systems: what it has meant for the clinician's understanding of pain and its treatment. *Pain,* 158(12): 2290-2300 (doi: 10.1097/j.pain.0000000000001043).

Baliki M. N., Apkarian A. V. (2015) Nociception, pain, negative moods, and behavior selection. *Neuron,* 87(3): 474-491 (doi: 10.1016/j.neuron.2015.06005).

Bannister K., Kucharczyk M., Dickenson A. H. (2017) Hopes for the future of pain control. *Pain Therapy,* 6(2): 117-128 (doi: 10.1007/s40122-017-0073-6).

Barbetta C., Currow D. C., Johnson M. J. (2017) Non-opioid medications for the relief of chronic breathlessness: current evidence. *Expert Rev Respir Med,* 11(4): 333-341 (doi: 10.1080/17476348.2017).

Basbaum A.I., Bautista D.M., Scherrer G., Julius D. (2009) Cellular and molecular mechanisms of pain. *Cell,* 139(2): 267-284 (doi: 10.1016/j.cell.2009.09.028).

Bastuji H., Frot M., Perchet C., Hagiwara K., Garcia-Larrea L. (2018) Convergence of sensory and limbic noxious input into the anterior insula and the emergence of pain from nociception. *Sci Rep,* 8(1): 13360 (doi: 10.1038/s41598-018-31781-z).

Benarroch E.E. (2019) Insular cortex: Functional complexity and clinical correlations. *Neurology,* 93(21): 932-938 (doi: 10.1212/WNL. 0000000000008525).

Bingel U., Tracey I. (2008) Imaging CNS modulation of pain in humans. *Physiology* (Bethesda), 23(6): 371-380 (doi: 10.1152/physiol.00024. 2008).

Bosier B., Muccioli G.G., Hermans E., Lambert D.M. (2010) Functionally selective cannabinoid receptor signaling: therapeutic implications and opportunities. *Biochem Pharmacol,* 80(1): 1-12 (doi: 10.1016/j.bcp. 2010.02.013).

Brooks J.C.W., Tracey I. (2007) The insula: A multidimensional integration site for pain. *Pain,* 128(1): 1–2 (doi: 10.1016/j.pain.2006.12.025).

Brown C.A., Matthews J., Fairclough M., McMahon A., Barnett E., Al-Kaysi A., El-Deredy W., Jones A.K. (2015) Striatal opioid receptor availability is related to acute and chronic pain perception in arthritis: Does opioid adaptation increase resilience to chronic pain? *Pain,* 156(11): 2267–2275 (doi: 10.1097/j.pain.0000000000000299).

Bushnell M. C., Ceko M., Low L. A. (2013) Cognitive and emotional control of pain and its disruption in chronic pain. *Nature Rev Neurosci,* 14(7): 502–511 (doi: 10.1038/nrn3516).

Cai Y.Q., Wang W., Paulucci-Holthauzen A., Pan Z.Z. (2018) Brain circuits mediating opposing effects on emotion and pain. *J Neurosci,* 38(28): 6340-6349 (doi: 10.1523/JNEUROSCI.2780-17.2018).

Casey K.L. (2000) Concepts of pain mechanisms: the contributions of functional imaging of the human brain. *Prog Brain Res,* 129: 277-287 (doi: 10.1016/S0079-6123(00)29020-1).

Chen Q., Heinricher M.M. (2019) Descending control mechanisms and chronic pain. *Curr Rheumatol Rep,* 21(5): 13 (doi: 10.1007/s11926-019-0813-1).

Console-Bram L., Marcu J., Abood M.E. (2012) Cannabinoid receptors: nomenclature and pharmacological principles. *Prog Neuropsychopharmacol Biol Psychiatry,* 38(1): 4-15 (doi: 10.1016/j.pnpbp.2012.02. 009).

Corkin S., Hebben N. (1981) Subjective estimates of chronic pain before and after psychosurgery or treatment in a pain unit. *Pain,* 11(Suppl. 1): S150 (doi: 10.1016/0304-3959(81)90390-0).

Costa-Pereira J. T., Serrão P., Martins I., Tavares I. (2020) Serotoninergic pain modulation from the rostral ventromedial medulla (RVM) in chemotherapy-induced neuropathy: The role of spinal 5-HT3 receptors. *Eur J Neurosci,* 51(8): 1756-1769 (doi: 10.1111/ejn.14614).

Craig A.D. (2011) Significance of the insula for the evolution of human awareness of feelings from the body. *Ann NY Acad Sci,* 1225: 72–82 (doi: 10.1111/j.1749-6632.2011.05990.x).

Craig A.D. (2014) Topographically organized projection to posterior insular cortex from the posterior portion of the ventral medial nucleus in the long-tailed macaque monkey. *J Comp Neurol,* 522(1): 36–63 (doi: 10.1002/cne.23425).

Craig K.D. (2006) Emotions and psychobiology. In: *Wall and Mellzack's Textbook of Pain,* 5th ed. S.B. McMahon, M. Koltzenburg (eds). London: Elsevier, pp. 231-240.

Cristino L., Bisogno T., Di Marzo V. (2020) Cannabinoids and the expanded endocannabinoid system in neurological disorders. *Nature Rev Neurol,* 16(1): 9-29 (doi: 10.1038/s41582-019-0284-z).

Cryer B., Barnett M.A., Wagner J., Wilcox C.M. (2016) Overuse and misperceptions of non-steroidal anti-inflammatory drugs in the United States. *Am J Med Sci,* 352(5): 472–480 (doi: 10.1016/j.amjms.2016.08.028).

Darcq E., Kieffer B.L. (2018) Opioid receptors: drivers to addiction? *Nature Rev Neurosci,* 19(8): 499–514 (doi: 10.1038/s41583-018-0028-x).

Da Silva J.T., Seminowicz D.A. (2019) Neuroimaging of pain in animal models: a review of recent literature. *Pain Rep,* 4(4): e732 (doi: 10.1097/PR9.0000000000000732).

Desroches J., Beaulieu P. (2010) Opioids and cannabinoids interactions: Involvement in pain management. *Curr Drug Targets,* 11(4): 462-473 (doi: 10.2174/138945010790980303).

Desroches J., Bouchard J. F., Gendron L., Beaulieu P. (2014) Involvement of cannabinoid receptors in peripheral and spinal morphine analgesia. *Neurosci,* 261: 23-42 (doi: 10.1016/j.neuroscience.2013.12.030).

Dickenson A.H., Kieffer B.L. (2013) Opioids: Basic mechanisms. In: *Wall and Melzack's Textbook of Pain.* 6th ed. S.B. McMahon et al. (eds). Chapter 30, Elsevier, pp. 413-428.

Di Marzo V. (2009) The endocannabinoid system: Its general strategy of action, tools for its pharmacological manipulation and potential therapeutic exploitation. *Pharmacol Res,* 60(2): 77-84 (doi: 10.1016/j.phrs.2009.02.010).

Di Marzo V. (2018) New approaches and challenges to targeting the endocannabinoid system. *Nature Rev Drug Discov,* 17(9): 623-639 (doi: 10.1038/nrd.2018.115).

Di Marzo V., Stella N., Zimmer A. (2015) Endocannabinoid signaling and the deteriorating brain. *Nature Rev Neurosci,* 16(1): 30-42 (doi: 10.1038/nrn3876).

Drake C.T., Chavkin C., Milner T.A. (2007) Opioid systems in the dentate gyrus. In: *The Dentate Gyrus: A Comprehensive Guide to Structure, Function, and Clinical Implications,* H. E. Scharfman (ed.). *Prog Brain Res,* 163: 245-263 (doi: 10.1016/S0079-6123(07) 63015-5).

Duric V., McCarson K.E., (2006) Persistent pain produces stress-like alterations in hippocampal neurogenesis and gene expression. *J Pain,* 7(8), 544–555 (doi: 10.1016/j.jpain.2006.01.458).

Duric V., McCarson K.E. (2007) Neurokinin-1 (NK-1) receptor and brain-derived neurotrophic factor (BDNF) gene expression is differentially modulated in the rat spinal dorsal horn and hippocampus during inflammatory pain. *Mol Pain,* 3: 32–40 (doi: 10.1186/1744-8069-3-32).

Eichenbaum H. (2017) Memory: Organization and control. *Annu Rev Psychol,* 68: 19–45 (doi: 10.1146/annurev-psych-010416-044131).

Elman I., Borsook D., Volkow N.D. (2013) Pain and suicidality: Insights from reward and addiction neuroscience. *Prog Neurobiol,* 109: 1–27 (doi: 10.1016/j.pneurobio.2013.06.003).

Escobar W., Ramirez K., Avila C., Limongi R., Vanegas H., Vazquez E. (2012) Metamizol, a non-opioid analgesic, acts via endocannabinoids in the PAG-RVM axis during inflammation in rats. *Eur J Pain,* 16(5): 676-689 (doi: 10. 1002/j.1532-2149.2011.00057.x).

Fasick V., Spengler R.N., Samankan S., Nader N.D., Ignatowski T.A. (2015) The hippocampus and TNF: Common links between chronic pain and depression. *Neurosci Biobehav Rev,* 53: 139-159 (doi: 10.1016/j.neubiorev.2015.03.014).

Favaroni Mendes L.A., Menescal-de-Oliveira L. (2008) Role of cholinergic, opioidergic and GABA-ergic neurotransmission of the dorsal hippocampus in the modulation of nociception in guinea pigs. *Life Science,* 83 (19-20): 644-650 (doi: 10.1016/j.lfs.2008.09.006).

Feinstein J.S., Khalsa S.S., Salomons T.V., Prkachin K.M., Frey-Law L.A., Lee J.E., Tranel D., Rudrauf D. (2016) Preserved emotional awareness of pain in a patient with extensive bilateral damage to the insula, anterior cingulate, and amygdala. *Brain Struct Funct*, 221: 1499–1511 (doi: 10.1007/s00429-014-0986-3).

Fields H.L. (2014) More pain; less gain. *Science*, 345(6196): 513–514 (doi: 10.1126/science.1258477).

Fishbain D.A., Lewis J.E., Gao J. (2014) The pain suicidality association: A narrative review. *Pain Med*, 15(11): 1835–1849 (doi: 10.1111/pme.12463).

Frot M., Faillenot I., Mauguière F. (2014) Processing of nociceptive input from posterior to anterior insula in humans. *Hum Brain Mapp*, 3(11): 5486–5499 (doi: 10.1002/hbm.22565).

Galhardoni R., Aparecida da Silva V., García-Larrea L., Dale C., Baptista A. F., Barbosa L.M., Menezes L.M.B., de Siqueira S.R.D.T., Valério F. et al. (2019) Insular and anterior cingulate cortex deep stimulation for central neuropathic pain: Disassembling the percept of pain. *Neurology*, 92(18): e2165-e2175 (doi: 10.1212 /WNL. 0000000000007396).

Gibson H. E., Edwards J. G., Page R. S., Van Hook M. J., Kauer J A. (2008) TRPV1 channels mediate long-term depression at synapses on hippocampal interneurons. *Neuron*, 57(5): 746-759 (doi: 10.1016/j.neuron.2007.12.027).

Guida F., Luongo L., Marmo F., Romano R., Iannotta M., Napolitano F., Belardo C., Marabese I. et al. (2015). Palmitoyl ethanolamide reduces pain-related behaviors and restores glutamatergic synapses homeostasis in the medial prefrontal cortex of neuropathic mice. *Mol Brain*, 8: art. 47 (doi: 10.1186/s13041-015-0139-5).

Guindon J., Hohmann A.G. (2008) Cannabinoid CB2 receptors: a therapeutic target for the treatment of inflammatory and neuropathic pain. *Brit J Pharmacol*, 153(2): 319–334 (doi: 10.1038/sj.bjp.0707531).

Gurtskaia G., Tsiklauri N., Nozadze I., Nebieridze M., Tsagareli M.G. (2014a) Antinociceptive tolerance effects of NSAIDs microinjected into dorsal hippocampus. *BMC Pharmacol Toxicol*, 15, art. 10 (doi: 10.1186/2050-6511-15-10).

Gurtskaia G., Tsiklauri N., Nozadze I., Tsagareli M.G. (2014b) An overview of antinociceptive tolerance to non-steroidal anti-inflammatory drugs. *Annu Res Review Biol*, 4(12): 1887-1901.

Haase J., Brown E. (2015) Integrating the monoamine, neurotrophin and cytokine hypotheses of depression – A central role for the serotonin transporter? *Pharmacol Ther,* 147(1): 1–11 (doi: 10.1016/j.pharmthera. 2014. 10.002).

Heinricher M. M., Fields H.L. (2013) Central nervous system mechanisms of pain modulation. In: *Wall & Melzack Textbook of Pain,* 6th edition, S.B. McMahon et al. (eds.), Elsevier, pp. 129-142.

Heinricher M.M., Ingram S.L. (2009) The brainstem and nociceptive modulation. In: A.I. Basbaum, M.C. Bushnell (eds.), *Science of Pain.* San Diego: Elsevier, pp. 593-626.

Hemington K.S., Coulombe M.A. (2015) The periaqueductal gray and descending pain modulation: Why should we study them and what role do they play in chronic pain? *J Neurophysiol,* 114(4): 2080–2083 (doi: 10.1152/jn.00998.2014).

Henderson L.A., Gandevia S.C., Macefield V.G. (2007) Somatotopic organization of the processing of muscle and cutaneous pain in the left and right insula cortex: A single-trial fMRI study. *Pain,* 128(1): 20–30 (doi: 10.1016/j.pain.2006.08.013).

Henssen D., Dijk J., Knepflé R., Sieffers M., Winter A., Vissers K. (2019) Alterations in grey matter density and functional connectivity in trigeminal neuropathic pain and trigeminal neuralgia: A systematic review and meta-analysis. *Neuroimage Clin,* 24: 102039 (doi: 10.1016/ j.nicl.2019.102039).

Hernández-Delgadillo G.P., Cruz S.L. (2006) Endogenous opioids are involved in morphine and dipyrone analgesic potentiation in the tail flick test in rats. *Eur J Pharmacol,* 546(1-3): 54-59 (doi: 10.1016/j.ejphar. 2006.07.027).

Hill K.P., Palastro M.D., Johnson B., Ditre J.W. (2017) Cannabis and pain: A clinical review. *Cannabis Cannabinoid Res,* 2(1): 96–104 (doi: 10. 1089/can.2017.0017).

Hohmann A.G., Rice A.S.C. (2013) Cannabinoids. In: *Wall and Melzack's Texbook of Pain.* S.B. McMahon et al. (eds), Elsevier, pp. 538-551.

Holden J.E, Jeong Y., Forrest J.M. (2005) The endogenous opioid system and clinical pain management. *AACN Clin Issues,* 16(3): 291-301 (doi: 10.1097/00044067-200507000-00003).

Holsteg G. (2014) The periaqueductal gray controls brainstem emotional motor systems including respiration. *Prog Brain Res,* 209: 379–405 (doi: 10.1016/B978-0-444-63274-6.00020-5).

Hou Y.Y., Cai Y.Q., Pan Z.Z. (2020) GluA1 in central amygdala promotes opioid use and reverses inhibitory effect of pain. *Neuroscience*, 426: 141-153 (doi: 10.1016/j.neuroscience.2019.11.032).

Ito T., Tanaka-Mizuno S., Iwashita N., Tooyama I., Shiino A., Miura K. et al. (2017) Proton magnetic resonance spectroscopy assessment of metabolite status of the anterior cingulate cortex in chronic pain patients and healthy controls. *J Pain Res,* 10: 287–293 (doi: 10.2147/JPR.S123403).

Jasmin L., Ohara P.T. (2009) The rostral agranular insular cortex. In: *Science of Pain.* A.I. Basbaum, M. C. Bushnell (eds). Oxford, Elsevier, pp. 717-722.

Jasmin L., Rabkin S.D., Granato A., Boudah A., Ohara P.T. (2003) Analgesia and hyperalgesia from GABA-mediated modulation of the cerebral cortex. *Nature,* 424(6946): 316–320 (doi: 10.1038/nature01808).

Jimenez X.F. (2018) Cannabis for chronic pain: Not a simple solution. *Cleveland Clin J Med,* 85(12): 950–952 (doi: 10.3949/ccjm.85a.18089).

Johansen J. P., Fields H.L. (2004) Glutamatergic activation of anterior cingulate cortex produces an aversive teaching signal. *Nature Neurosci*, 7(4): 398-403 (doi: 10.1038/nn1207).

Johansen J.P., Fields H.L., Manning B.H. (2001) The affective component of pain in rodents: Direct evidence for a contribution of the anterior cingulate cortex. *PNAS,* 98(14): 8077–8082 (doi: 10.1073/pnas.141218998).

Kang D., McAuley J.H., Kassem M.S., Gatt J.M., Gustin S.M. (2019) What does the grey matter decrease in the medial prefrontal cortex reflect in people with chronic pain? *Eur J Pain,* 23(2): 203–219 (doi: 10.1002/ejp.1304).

Kato F., Sugimura Y.K., Takahashi Y. (2018) Pain-associated neural plasticity in the parabrachial to central amygdala circuit. In: *Advances in Pain Research: Mechanisms and Modulation of Chronic Pain.* B.-C. Shyu, M. Tominaga (eds.), Springer Nature, *Adv Exp Med Biol,* 1099: 157-166 (doi: 10.1007/978-981-13-1756-9_14).

Kazantzis N.P., Casey S.L., Seow P.W., Mitchell V.A., Vaughan C.W. (2016) Opioid and cannabinoid synergy in a mouse neuropathic pain model. *British J Pharmacol,* 173(16): 2521-2531 (doi: 10.1111/bph.13534).

Keay K., Bandler R. (2009) Emotional and behavioral significance of the pain signal and the role of the midbrain periaqueductal gray (PAG). In:

Science of Pain, A.I. Basbaum & M.C. Bushnell, (eds). Elsevier, San Diego, CA, pp. 627–634.

Khasabova I.A., Gielissen J., Chandiramani A., Harding-Rose C., Odeh D. A., Simone D.A., Seybold V.S. (2011) CB1 and CB2 receptor agonists promote analgesia through synergy in a murine model of tumor pain. *Behavioural Pharmacol,* 22(5-6): 607–616 (doi: 10.1097/FBP. 0b013e3283474a6d).

Kmietowicz, Z. (2010) Cannabis based drug is licensed for spasticity in patients with MS. *BMJ* 340, c3363 (doi: 10.1136/bmj.c3363).

Koltzenburg M., Wall P.D., McMahon S.B. (1999) Does the right side know what the left is doing? *Trends Neurosci,* 22(3): 122-127 (doi: 10.1016/s0166-2236(98)01302-2).

Krebs M.O., Kebir O., Jay T.M. (2019) Exposure to cannabinoids can lead to persistent cognitive and psychiatric Disorders. *Eur J Pain,* 23(7): 1225-1233 (doi: 10.1002/ejp.1377).

Kuner R, Flor H. (2017) Structural plasticity and reorganisation in chronic pain. *Nature Rev Neurosci,* 18(1): 20-30 (doi: 10.1038/nrn.2016.162).

Lane D.A., Patel P.A., Morgan M.M. (2005) Evidence for an intrinsic mechanism of antinociceptive tolerance within the ventrolateral periaqueductal gray of rats. *Neurosci,* 135(1): 227-234 (doi: 10.1016/j.neuroscience.2005.06.014).

Lathe R. (2001) Hormones and the hippocampus. *J Endocrinol,* 169(2): 205–231 (doi: 10.1677/joe.0.1690205).

Lau B.K., Vaughan C.W. (2014a) Targeting the endogenous cannabinoid system to treat neuropathic pain. *Frontiers Pharmacol* 5(3), art. 28 (doi: 10.3389/fphar.2014.00028).

Lau B.K, Vaughan C.W. (2014b) Descending modulation of pain: the GABA disinhibition hypothesis of analgesia. *Current Opin Neurobiol,* 29: 159–164 (doi: 10.1016/j.conb.2014.07.010).

Lau B.K., Winters B.L., Vaughan CW. (2020) Opioid presynaptic disinhibition of the midbrain periaqueductal grey descending analgesic pathway. *British J Pharmacol,* 177(10): 2320-2332 (doi: 10.1111/bph.14982).

Leknes S., Tracey I. (2008) A common neurobiology for pain and pleasure. *Nature Rev Neurosci,* 9(6), 314–320 (doi: 10.1038/ nrn2333).

Li J.X. (2019) Combining opioids and non-opioids for pain management: Current status. *Neuropharmacol.,* 158: art. 107619 (doi: 10.1016/j.neuropharm.2019.04.025).

Lichtman A.H., Martin B.R. (2005) Cannabinoid tolerance and dependence. *Handb Exp Pharmacol.,* 168: 691-717 (doi: 10.1007/3-540-26573-2_24)

Liu L.Y., Zhang R.L., Chen L., Zhao H.Y., Cai J., Wang J.K., Guo D.Q., Cui Y.J., Xing G.G. (2019) Chronic stress increases pain sensitivity via activation of the rACC-BLA pathway in rats. *Exp Neurol*, 313: 109-123 (doi: 10.1016/j.expneurol.2018.12.009).

Liu M.G., Chen J. (2009) Roles of the hippocampal formation in pain information processing. *Neurosci Bull*, 25(5): 237-266 (doi: 10.1007/s12264-009-0905-4).

Liu M.G., Kang S.J., Shi T.Y., Koga K., Zhang M.M., Collingridge G.L., Kaang B.K., Zhuo M. (2013) Long-term potentiation of synaptic transmission in the adult mouse insular cortex: multielectrode array recordings. *J Neurophysiol*, 110(2): 505–521 (doi: 10.1152/jn.01104.2012).

Llorca-Torralba M., Suarez-Pereira I., Bravo L., Camarena-Delgado C., Garcia-Partida J.A., Mico J.A., Berrocoso E. (2019) Chemogenetic silencing of the Locus Coeruleus-Basolateral Amygdala pathway abolishes pain-induced anxiety and enhanced aversive learning in rats. *Biol Psychiatry*, 85(12): 1021–1035 (doi: 10.1016/j.biopsych.2019.02.018).

Lötsch J., Weyer-Menkhoff I., Tegeder I. (2018) Current evidence of cannabinoid-based analgesia obtained in preclinical and human experimental settings. *Eur J Pain*, 22(3): 471–484 (doi: 10.1002/ejp.1148).

Lu C., Yang T., Zhao H., Zhang M., Meng F., Fu H., Xie Y., Xu H. (2016) Insular cortex is critical for the perception, modulation, and chronification of pain. *Neurosci Bull*, 32(2):191-201 (doi:10.1007/s12264-016-0016-y).

Luongo L., Starowicz K., Maione S., Di Marzo V. (2017) Allodynia lowering induced by cannabinoids and endocannabinoids (ALICE). *Pharmacol Res*, 119: 272-277 (doi: 10.1016/j.phrs.2017.02.019).

Lutz P.E., Kieffer B.L. (2013) Opioid receptors: distinct roles in mood disorders. *Trends Neurosci*, 36(3): 195–206 (doi: 10.1016/j.tins.2012.11.002).

Macey T.A, Bobeck E.N., Suchland K.L., Morgan M.M., Ingram S.L. (2015) Change in functional selectivity of morphine with the development of antinociceptive tolerance. *Brit J Pharmacol*, 172(2): 549-561 (doi: 10.1111/bph.12703).

MacLean P.D. (1952) Some psychiatric implications of physiological studies on frontotemporal portion of limbic system (visceral brain). *EEG Clin Neurophysiol*, 4(4): 407-418 (doi: 10.1016/0013-4694(52)90073-4).

Maguire D.R., France C.P. (2016) Interactions between cannabinoid receptor agonists and mu opioid receptor agonists in rhesus monkeys discriminating fentanyl. *Eur J Pharmacol,* 784: 199-206 (doi: 10.1016/j.ejphar.2016.05.018).

Malmberg A.B., Yaksh T.L. (1992) Antinociceptive actions of spinal nonsteroidal anti-inflammatory agents on the formalin test in the rat. *J Pharmacol Exp Ther,* 263(1): 136–146.

Maldonado R., Banos J.E., Cabanero D. (2016) The endocannabinoid system and neuropathic pain. *Pain,* 157(2) Suppl. 1: S23-S32 (doi: 10.1097/j.pain.0000000000000428).

Maletic V., Robinson M., Oakes T., Iyengar S., Ball S. G., Russell, J. (2007) Neurobiology of depression: an integrated view of key findings. *Int J Clin Pract,* 61(12): 2030–2040 (doi: 10.1111/j.1742-1241.2007. 01602.x).

Mallipeddi S., Janero D.R., Zvonok N., Makriyannis A. (2017) Functional selectivity at G-protein coupled receptors: Advancing cannabinoid receptors as drug targets. *Biochem Pharmacol,* 128: 1-11 (doi: 10.1016/j.bcp.2016).

Mansour A.R., Farmer M.A., Baliki M.N., Apkarian A.V. (2014) Chronic pain: The role of learning and brain plasticity. *Restor Neurol Neurosci,* 32(1): 129–139 (doi: 10.3233/RNN-139003).

Mastinu A., Premoli M., Ferrari-Toninelli G., Tambaro S., Maccarinelli G., Memo M., Bonini S.A. (2018). Cannabinoids in health and disease: pharmacological potential in metabolic syndrome and neuroinflammation. *Horm Mol Biol Clin Investig,* 36(2): 0013 (doi: 10.1515/hmbci-2018-0013).

Mazzola L., Isnard J., Peyron R., Guénot M., Mauguière F. (2009) Somatotopic organization of pain responses to direct electrical stimulation of the human insular cortex. *Pain,* 146(1): 99–104 (doi: 10.1016/j.pain.2009. 07.014).

Mechoulam R. (2019) The pharmacohistory of cannabis sativa. In: *Cannabinoids as Therapeutic Agents.* R. Mechoulam (ed.). Chapter 1, Boca Renton: Chapman & Hall/CRC Press, pp. 1-20.

Moore A., McQuay H.J. (2013) Cyclooxygenase inhibitors: Clinical use. In: *Wall and Melzack's Textbook of Pain,* 6th ed., S. B. McMahon et al. (eds.), chap. 33. Philadelphia: Elsevier-Saunders, pp: 455-464.

Morales P., Reggio P.H., Jagerovic N. (2017) An overview on medicinal chemistry of synthetic and natural derivatives of cannabidiol. *Front Pharmacol,* 8: 422 (doi: 10.3389/fphar.2017.00422).

Morris L.S., Sprenger C., Koda K., de la Mora D.M., Yamada T., Mano H., Kashiwagi Y., Yoshioka Y., Morioka Y., Seymour B. (2018) Anterior cingulate cortex connectivity is associated with suppression of behavior in a rat model of chronic pain. *Brain Neurosci Adv*, 2: 1–7 (doi: 10.1177/ 2398212818779646).

Mun C.J., Letzen J.E., Peters E.N., Campbell C.M., Vandrey R., Gajewski-Nemes J. et al. (2020) Cannabinoid effects on responses to quantitative sensory testing among individuals with and without clinical pain: a systematic review. *Pain*, 161(2): 244-260 (doi: 10.1097/j.pain. 0000000000001720).

Mutso A.A., Radzicki D., Baliki M.N., Huang L., Banisadr G., Centeno M.V. et al. (2012) Abnormalities in hippocampal functioning with persistent pain. *J Neurosci*, 32(17): 5747-5756 (doi: 10.1523/JNEUROSCI.0587-12.2012).

Mücke M., Phillips T., Radbruch L., Petzke F., Häuser W. (2018) Cannabis-based medicines for chronic neuropathic pain in adults. *Cochrane Database System Rev*, 3, art: CD012182 (doi: 10.1002/14651858. CD012182.pub2).

McCarberg B., Peppin J. (2019) Pain pathways and nervous system plasticity: Learning and memory in pain. *Pain Med*, 20(12): 2421-2437 (doi: 10.1093/pm/pnz017).

McCrae C.S., O'Shea A.M., Boissoneault J., Vatthauer K.E., Robinson M.E., Staud R., Perlstein W.M., Craggs J.G. (2015) Fibromyalgia patients have reduced hippocampal volume compared with healthy controls. *J Pain Res*, 8: 47-52 (doi: 10.2147/JPR.S71959).

McEwen B.S. (2001) Plasticity of the hippocampus: adaptation to chronic stress and allostatic load. *Ann NY Acad Sci* 933: 265–277 (doi: 10.1111/ j.1749-6632.2001.tb05830.x).

McKenna J.E., Melzack R. (1992) Analgesia produced microinjection in dentate gyrus. *Pain*, 49(1): 105-112 (doi: 10. 1016/0304-3959(92) 90195-h).

Nadal X., La Porta C., Bura S.A., Maldonado R. (2013) Involvement of the opioid and cannabinoid systems in pain control: New insights from knockout studies. *Eur J Pharmacol*, 716(1-3): 142-157 (doi: 10.1016/j. ejphar.2013.01.077).

Natura G., Bär K. J., Eitner A., Boettger M. K., Richter F., Hensellek S., et al. (2013) Neuronal prostaglandin E2 receptor subtype EP3 mediates antinociception during inflammation. *Proc Natl Acad Sci USA*, 110: 13648–13653 (doi: 10. 1073/pnas.1300820110).

Navratilova E., Atcherley C.W., Porreca F. (2015) Brain circuits encoding reward from pain relief. *Trends Neurosci,* 38 (11): 741–750 (doi: 10.1016/j.tins.2015.09.003).

Navratilova E., Ji G., Phelps C., Qu C., Hein M., Yakhnitsa V., Neugebauer V., Porreca F. (2019) Kappa opioid signaling in the central nucleus of the amygdala promotes disinhibition and aversiveness of chronic neuropathic pain. *Pain,* 160(4): 824-832 (doi: 10.1097/j.pain.0000000000001458).

Navratilova E., Nation K., Remeniuk B., Neugebauer V., Bannister K., Dickenson A.H., Porreca F. (2020) Selective modulation of tonic aversive qualities of neuropathic pain by morphine in the central nucleus of the amygdala requires endogenous opioid signaling in the anterior cingulate cortex. *Pain,* 161(3): 609-618 (doi: 10.1097/j.pain.0000000000001748).

Navratilova E., Xie J. Y., Meske D., Qu C., Morimura K., Okun A., Arakawa N. et al. (2015) Endogenous opioid activity in the anterior cingulate cortex is required for relief of pain. *J Neurosci,* 35(18): 7264–7271 (doi: 10.1523 /JNEUROSCI.3862-14.2015).

Neugebauer V. (2015) Amygdala pain mechanisms. *Handb Exp Pharmacol,* 227: 261–284 (doi: 10.1007/978-3-662-46450-2_13).

Nevian T. (2017) The cingulate cortex: divided in pain. *Nature Neurosci,* 20(11): 1515-1517 (doi: 10.1038/nn.4664).

Nielsen S., Sabioni P., Trigo J.M., Ware M.A., Betz-Stablein B.D., Murnion B., Lintzeris N., Khor K.E. et al. (2017) Opioid-sparing effect of cannabinoids: A systematic review and meta-analysis. *Neuropsychopharmacol,* 42(9): 1752-1765 (doi: 10.1038/npp.2017.51).

Nieuwenhuys R. (2012) The insular cortex: A review. In: *Evolution of the Primate Brain.* M.A. Hofman, D. Falk (eds.), Elsevier. Chap. 7. *Prog Brain Res,* 195: 123-163 (doi: 10.1016/B978-0-444-53860-4.00007-6).

Ohara P.T., Granato A., Moallem T.M., Wang B.R., Tillet Y., Jasmin L. (2003) Dopaminergic input to GABA-ergic neurons in the rostral agranular insular cortex of the rat. *J Neurocytol,* 32(2): 131–141 (doi: 10.1023/ b:neur.0000005598.09647.7f).

Okine B.N., Rea K., Olango W.M., Price J., Herdman S., Madasu M.K., Roche M., Finn D.P. (2014) A role for PPAR alpha in the medial prefrontal cortex in formalin-evoked nociceptive responding in rats. *Brit J Pharmacol,* 171: 1462–1471 (doi: 10.1111/bph.12540).

Okine B.N, Madasu M.K., McGowan F., Prendergast C., Gaspar J.C., Harhen B., Roche M., Finn D.P. (2016) N-palmitoylethanolamide in the anterior cingulate cortex attenuates inflammatory pain behavior indirectly via a CB1 receptor-mediated mechanism. *Pain,* 157(12): 2687-2696 (doi: 10.1097/j.pain.0000000000000687).

Okine B.N, Gaspar J.C., Finn D.P. (2019) PPARs and pain. *Brit J Pharmacol,* 176(10): 1421-1442 (doi: 10. 1111/bph.14339).

Ossipov M.H., Dussor G.O., Porreca F. (2010) Central modulation of pain. *J Clin Invest,* 120(11): 3779-3787 (doi: 10. 1172/JCI43766).

Ossipov M.H., Morimura K., Porreca F. (2014) Descending pain modulation and chronification of pain. *Curr Opin Support Palliat Care,* 8(2): 143–151 (doi: 10.1097/SPC.0000000000000055).

Palermo S., Benedetti F., Costa T., Amanzio M. (2015) Pain anticipation: an activation likelihood estimation meta-analysis of brain imaging studies. *Hum Brain Mapp,* 36(5): 1648–1661 (doi: 10.1002/hbm.22727).

Papez J.W. (1937) A proposed mechanism of emotion. *Arch Neurol Psychiat,* (Chicago), 38: 725-743.

Paxinos G., Watson C. (1997) *The Rat Brain in Stereotaxic Coordinates.* Compact 3rd ed. San Diego, CA: Academic Press.

Pecina M., Karp J.F., Mathew S., Todtenkopf M.S., Ehrich E.W., Zubieta J.K. (2019) Endogenous opioid system dysregulation in depression: implications for new therapeutic approaches. *Mol Psychiatry,* 24(4): 576-587 (doi: 10.1038 /s41380-018-0117-2).

Pernia-Andrade A.J., Tortorici V., Venegas H. (2004) Induction of opioid tolerance by lysine acetylsalicylate in rats. *Pain,* 111(1/2): 191-200 (doi: 10.1016/j.pain.2004.06.006).

Pert C.B., Snyder S.H. (1973) Opiate receptor: demonstration in nervous tissue. *Science,* 179(4077): 1011–1014 (doi: 10.1126/science.179. 4077.1011).

Pertwee R.G., Howlett A.C., Abood M.E., Alexander S.P., Di Marzo V. et al. (2010) Cannabinoid receptors and their ligands: beyond CB1 and CB2. *Pharmacol Rev,* 62: 588–631 (doi: 10.1124/pr.110.003004).

Petzke F., Klose P., Welsch P., Sommer C., Häuser W. (2020) Opioids for chronic low back pain: An updated systematic review and meta-analysis of efficacy, tolerability and safety in randomized placebo-controlled studies of at least 4 weeks of double-blind duration. *Eur J Pain,* 24(3): 497-517 (doi: 10.1002/ejp.1519).

Piomelli D., Sass, O. (2014) Peripheral gating of pain signals by endogenous lipid mediators. *Nature Neurosci,* 17(2): 164–174 (doi: 10.1038/nn. 3612).

Pirkulashvili N., Tsiklauri N., Nebieridze M., Tsagareli M.G. (2017) Antinociceptive tolerance to NSAIDs in the agranular insular cortex is mediated by opioid mechanism. *J Pain Res,* 10: 1561–1568 (doi: 10.2147/JPR.S138360).

Prescott S.A., Ma Q., De Koninck Y. (2014) Normal and abnormal coding of somatosensory stimuli causing pain. *Nature Neurosci,* 17(2): 183–191 (doi: 10.1038/nn.3629).

Qiu S., Chen T., Koga K., Guo Y. Y., Xu H., Song Q., et al. (2013) An increase in synaptic NMDA receptors in the insular cortex contributes to neuropathic pain. *Sci Signal* 6(275): ra34 (doi: 10.1126/scisignal.2003778).

Qiu S., Zhang M., Liu Y., Guo Y., Zhao H., Song Q., et al. (2014) GluA1 phosphorylation contributes to postsynaptic amplification of neuropathic pain in the insular cortex. *J Neurosci,* 34(40): 13505–13515 (doi: 10.1523/jneurosci.1431-14.2014).

Racine M. (2018) Chronic pain and suicide risk: A comprehensive review. *Prog Neuro-Psychopharmacol Biol Psychiatry,* 87(Pt B): 269–280 (doi: 10.1016/j.pnpbp.2017.08.020).

Rance M., Ruttorf M., Nees F., Schad L. R., Flor H. (2014) Neurofeedback of the difference in activation of the anterior cingulate cortex and posterior insular cortex: two functionally connected areas in the processing of pain. *Front Behav Neurosci,* 8: 357 (doi: 10.3389/fnbeh.2014.00357).

Ren K., Dubner R. (2009) Descending control mechanisms. In: A.I., Basbaum, M.C. Bushnell (eds.), *Science of Pain.* San Diego: Elsevier, pp. 723-762.

Rubino T., Zamberletti E., Parolaro D. (2015) Endocannabinoids and mental disorders. In: *Endocannabinoids.* R. Pertwee (ed.). *Handb Exp Pharmacol,* Springer, 231: 261-283 (doi: 10.1007/978-3-319-20825 1_9).

Russo E., Guy G.W. (2006) A tale of two cannabinoids: the therapeutic rational for combining tetrahydro-cannabinol and cannabidiol. *Med Hypotheses,* 66(2): 234–246 (10.1016/j.mehy.2005.08.026).

Salas R., Ramirez K., Tortorici V., Vanegas H., Vazquez E. (2018) Functional relationship between brainstem putative pain-facilitating neurons and spinal nociceptive neurons during development of inflammation in rats. *Brain Res,* 1686: 55-64 (doi: 10.1016/j.brainres.2018.02.025).

Salas R., Ramirez K., Vanegas H., Vazquez E. (2016) Activity correlations between on-like and off-like cells of the rostral ventromedial medulla and simultaneously recorded wide-dynamic-range neurons of the spinal dorsal horn in rats. *Brain Res,* 1652: 103-110 (doi: 10.1016/j.brainres. 2016.10.001).

Sandkühler J. (2009) Models and mechanisms of hyperalgesia and allodynia. *Physiol Rev,* 89(2):707–758 (doi: 10.1152/physrev.00025. 2008).

Scavone J. L, Sterling R. C., Van Bockstaele E. J. (2013) Cannabinoid and opioid interactions: implications for opiate dependence and withdrawal. *Neuroscience,* 248: 637-654 (doi: 10.1016/j.neuroscience.2013.04. 034).

Schmidt B.L., Hamamoto D.T., Simone D.A., Wilcox G.L. (2010) Mechanism of cancer pain. *Molec Interv,* 10(3): 164-178 (doi: 10.1124/mi.10.3.7).

Schüchen R.H., Mücke M., Marinova M., Kravchenko D., Häuser W., Radbruch L., Conrad R. (2018) Systematic review and meta-analysis on non-opioid analgesics in palliative medicine. *J Cachexia Sarcopenia Muscle,* 9(7): 1235-1254 (doi: 10.1002/jcsm.12352).

Segerdahl A.R., Mezue M., Okell T.W., Farrar J.T., Tracey I. (2015) The dorsal posterior insula subserves a fundamental role in human pain. *Nature Neurosci,* 18(4): 499-503 (doi: 10.1038/nn.3969).

Seno M.D.J., Assis D.V., Gouveia F., Antunes G.F., Kuroki M., Oliveira C.C. et al. (2018) The critical role of amygdala subnuclei in nociceptive and depressive-like behaviors in peripheral neuropathy. *Sci Rep,* 8(1): 13608 (doi: 10.1038/s41598-018-31962-w).

Seibert K., Zhang Y., Leahy K., Hauser S., Masferrer J., Perkins W. et al. (1994) Pharmacological and biochemical demonstration of the role of cyclooxygenase 2 in inflammation and pain. *Proc Natl Acad Sci USA,* 91(25): 12013–12017 (doi:10.1073/pnas.91.25.12013).

Seymour B., Dolan R.J. (2013) Emotion, motivation and pain. In: *Wall and Melzack's Texbook of Pain*. S.B. McMahon et al. (eds), Elsevier, pp. 248-255.

Sheng J., Liu S., Wang Y., Cui R., Zhang X. (2017) The link between depression and chronic pain: Neural mechanisms in the brain. *Neural Plasticity,* 2017: 9724371 (doi: 10.1155/2017/9724371).

Simons L.E., Moulton E.A., Linnman C., Carpino E., Becerra L., Borsook D. (2014) The human amygdala and pain: Evidence from neuroimaging. *Hum Brain Mapp,* 35(2): 527–538 (doi: 10.1002/hbm.22199).

Sirohi S., Tiwari A. (2016) Pain in the management of opioid use disorder. *J Pain Res,* 9: 963–966 (doi: 10.2147/JPR.S123667).

Skolnick P. (2018) The opioid epidemic: Crisis and solutions. *Annu Rev Pharmacol Toxicol,* 58: 143–159 (doi: 10.1146/annurev-pharmtox 010617-052534).

Soliman N., Hohmann A.G., Haroutounian S., Wever K., Rice A.S.C., Finn D.P. (2019) A protocol for the systematic review and meta-analysis of studies in which cannabinoids were tested for antinociceptive effects in animal models of pathological or injury-related persistent pain. *Pain Rep,* 4(4): e766 (doi: 10.1097/PR9.0000000000000766).

Sommer C., Klose P., Welsch P., Petzke F., Häuser W. (2020) Opioids for chronic non-cancer neuropathic pain. An updated systematic review and meta-analysis of efficacy, tolerability and safety in randomized placebo-controlled studies of at least 4 weeks duration. *Eur J Pain,* 24(1): 3-18 (doi: 10.1002/ejp.1494).

Starowicz K., Finn D.P. (2017) Cannabinoids and pain: Sites and mechanisms of action. *Adv Pharmacol,* 80: 437–475 (doi: 10.1016/ bs.apha.2017.05.003).

Tan L.L., Pelzer P., Heinl C., Tang W., Gangadharan V., Flor H. et al. (2017) A pathway from midcingulate cortex to posterior insula gates nociceptive hypersensitivity. *Nature Neurosci,* 20(11): 1591-1601 (doi: 10.1038/nn.4645).

Tasker R.A.R., Choiniere M., Libman S.M., Melzack R. (1987) Analgesia produced by injection of lidocaine into the lateral hypothalamus. *Pain,* 31(2): 237-248 (doi: 10.1016/0304-3959(87)90039-x).

Telleria-Diaz A., Schmidt M., Kreusch S., Neubert A.K., Schache F., Vazquez E. et al. (2010) Spinal antinociceptive effects of cyclo-oxygenase inhibition during inflammation: Involvement of prostaglandins and endocannabinoids. *Pain,* 148(1): 26-35 (doi: 10.1016/j.pain.2009.08.013).

Thompson J.M., Neugebauer V. (2017) Amygdala plasticity and pain. *Pain Res Manag;* 2017: 8296501 (doi: 10.1155/2017/8296501).

Thompson J.M., Neugebauer V. (2019) Cortico-limbic pain mechanisms. *Neurosci Letters,* 702: 15-23 (doi: 10.1016/j.neulet.2018.11.037).

Topuz R.D, Gündüz Ö, Karadağ C.H., Dokmeci D., Ulugol A. (2019) Endocannabinoid and N-acylethanolamide levels in rat brain and spinal cord following systemic dipyrone and paracetamol administration. *Can J Physiol Pharmacol,* 97(11): 1035-1041 (doi: 10.1139/cjpp-2019-0015).

Topuz R.D., Gündüz Ö., Karadağ C.H., Ulugöl A. (2020) Non-opioid analgesics and the endocannabinoid system. *Balkan Med J*, 37(6): 309-315 (doi: 10.4274/balkanmedj.galenos.2020.2020.6.66).

Tortorici V., Aponte Y., Acevedo H., Nogueira L., Vanegas H. (2009) Tolerance to non-opioid analgesics in PAG involves unresponsiveness of medullary pain-modulating neurons in male rats. *Eur J Neurosci*, 29(6): 1188–1196 (doi: 10.1111/j.1460-9568.2009.06678.x).

Tortorici V., Nogueira L., Aponte Y., Vanegas H. (2004) Involvement of cholecystokinin in the opioid tolerance induced by dipyrone (metamizol) microinjections into the periaqueductal gray matter of rats. *Pain*, 112(1-2): 113–120 (doi:10.1016/j.pain.2004.08.006).

Tortorici V., Nogueira L., Salas R., Vanegas H. (2003) Involvement of local cholecystokinin in the tolerance induced by morphine microinjections into the periaqueductal gray of rats. *Pain*, 102(1-2): 9–16 (doi: 10.1016/s0304-3959 (02)00153-7).

Tortorici V., Vanegas H. (2000) Opioid tolerance induced by metamizol (dipyrone) microinjections into the periaqueductal gray of rats. *Eur J Neurosci*, 12(11): 4074–4080 (doi: 10.1046/j.1460-9568.2000.00295.x).

Tsagareli M.G. (2012) Pain concept and treatment by opioids: Historic review. In: *Opioids: Pharmacology, Clinical Uses and Adverse Effects*. Chapter 2. New York: Nova Science, pp. 15-33.

Tsagareli MG. (2013) Pain and memory: Do they share similar mechanisms. *World J Neurosci*, 3(1): 39-48 (doi: 10.4236/wjns.2013.31005).

Tsagareli M.G. (2018) *Pain Concept and Treatment: from Alkmaeon to Patrick Wall*. Lambert Acad. Publishing.

Tsagareli M.G, Nozadze I., Tsiklauri N., Gurtskaia G. (2011) Tolerance to non-opioid analgesics is opioid sensitive in the nucleus raphe magnus. *Front Neurosci*, 5: art. 92 (doi:10.3389/fnins.2011.00092).

Tsagareli M.G., Tsiklauri N.D., Gurtskaia G.P., Nozadze I.R., Abzianidze E.V. (2009) Tolerance effects induced by NSAIDs micro-injections into the central nucleus of the amygdala in rats. *Neurophysiol* (Springer), 41(6): 404– 408.

Tsagareli M.G., Tsiklauri N., Gurtskaia G., Nozadze I., Abzianidze E. (2010) The central nucleus of amygdala is involved in tolerance to the antinociceptive effect of NSAIDs. *Health*, 2(1): 64–68.

Tsagareli M.G., Tsiklauri N. (2012) *Behavioral Study of 'Non-Opioid Tolerance'*. New York: Nova Biomedical.

Tsagareli M.G., Tsiklauri N., Nozadze I., Gurtskaia G. (2012) Tolerance effects of NSAIDs microinjected into central amygdala, periaqueductal

grey, and nucleus raphe: Possible cellular mechanism. *Neural Regen Res*, **7**(13): 1029-1039 (doi: 10.3969/j.issn.1673-5374.2012.13.010).
Tsiklauri N.D., Nozadze I.R., Gurtskaia G.P., Tsagareli M.G. (2011) Opioid sensitivity of analgesia induced by microinjections of non-steroidal anti-inflammatory drugs into the nucleus raphe magnus. *Neurophysiol* (Springer), 43 (3): 213–216.
Tsiklauri N., Nozadze I., Gurtskaia G., Tsagareli M.G. (2017) Antinociceptive tolerance to NSAIDs in the rat formalin test is mediated by the opioid mechanism. *Pharmacol Reports,* 69(1): 168-175 (doi: 10.1016/j.pharep.2016.10.004).
Tsiklauri N., Nozadze I., Pirkulashvili N., Gurtskaia G., Nebieridze M., Abzianidze E., Tsagareli M.G. (2016). Cellular mechanisms of antinociceptive tolerance to non-steroidal anti-inflammatory drugs. In: *Systemic, Cellular and Molecular Mechanisms of Physiological Functions and Their Disorders.* Vol. 1, chap. 26. New York: Nova Biomedical, pp. 339-362.
Tsiklauri N., Pirkulashvili N., Nozadze I., Nebieridze M., Gurtskaia G., Abzianidze E., Tsagareli M.G. (2018a). Antinociceptive tolerance to NSAIDs in the anterior cingulate cortex is mediated via endogenous opioid mechanism. *BMC Pharmacol Toxicol,* 19(1): art. 2 (doi: 10.1186/s40360-017-0193-y).
Tsiklauri N., Pirkulashvili N., Nozadze I., Tsagareli N., Nebieridze M., Gurtskaia G., Abzianidze E., Tsagareli M. G. (2018b) Brain limbic areas involved in the tolerance of NSAIDs via opioid mechanism. In: *Systemic, Cellular and Molecular Mechanisms of Physiological Functions and Their Disorders.* Vol. 2, chap. 23. New York: Nova, pp. 281-301.
Tsiklauri N., Tsagareli M.G. (2006) Non-opioid-induced tolerance in rats. *Neurophysiol* (Springer), 38(4): 370-373.
Tsiklauri N., Viatchenko-Karpinski V., Voitenko N., Tsagareli M.G. (2009) Non-opioid tolerance in juvenile and adult rats. *Eur J Pharmacol,* 629(1-3): 68-72 (doi: 10.1016/j.ejphar.2009.12.016).
Vaccarino A.L., Melzack R. (1989) Analgesia produced by injection of lidocaine into the anterior cingulum bundle of the rat. *Pain,* 39(2): 213-219 (doi: 10.1016/0304-3959(89)90008-0).
Vachon-Presseau E., Centen M. V., Ren W., Berger S. E., Tetreault P., Ghantous M. et al. (2016). The emotional brain as a predictor and amplifier of chronic pain. *J Dent Res*, 95(6): 605–612 (doi: 10.1177/0022034516638027).

Valentino R.J., Volkow N.D. (2018) Untangling the complexity of opioid receptor function. *Neuropsycho-pharmacol,* 43(13): 2514-2520 (doi: 10.1038/s41386-018-0225-3).

Vanegas H., Schaible H. G. (2001) Prostaglandins and cyclooxygenases in the spinal cord. *Prog Neurobiol,* 64(4): 327–363 (doi: 10.1016/s0301-0082(00)00063-0).

Vanegas H., Tortorici V. (2002) Opioidergic effects of non-opioid analgesics on the central nervous system. *Cell Mol Neurobiol,* 22(5-6): 655-661 (doi: 10.1023/a:1021896622089).

Vanegas H., Tortorici V. (2007). The periaqueductal gray as critical site for antinociception and tolerance induced by non-steroidal antiinflammatory drugs. In: S. Maione, V. Di Marzo (eds.). *Neurotransmission Antinociceptive Descending Pathway.* Kerala: Research Signpost, pp. 69-80.

Vanegas H., Vazquez E., Tortorici V. (2010) NSAIDs, opioids, cannabinoids and the control of pain by the central nervous system. *Pharmaceuticals,* 3: 1335–1347 (doi: 10.3390/ph3051335).

Vazquez E., Hernandez N., Escobar W., Vanegas H. (2005) Antinociception induced by intravenous dipyrone (metamizole) upon dorsal horn neurons: involvement of endogenous opioids at the periaqueductal gray matter, the nucleus raphe magnus, and the spinal cord in rats. *Brain Res,* 1048 (1-2): 211–217 (doi: 10.1016/j.brainres.2005.04.083).

Vazquez E., Escobar W., Ramirez C., Vanegas H. (2007) A non-opioid analgesic acts upon the PAG-RVM axis to reverse inflammatory hyperalgesia. *Eur J Neurosci,* 25(2): 471-479 (doi: 10.1111/j.1460-9568.2007.05280.x).

Volkers R., Giesen E., van der Heiden M., Kerperien M., Lange S., Kurt E. et al. (2020) Invasive motor cortex stimulation influences intracerebral structures in patients with neuropathic pain: An activation likelihood estimation meta-analysis of imaging data. *Neuromodulation,* 23(4): 436-443 (doi: 10.1111/ner.13119).

Vuilleumier P.H., Schliessbach J., Curatolo M. (2018) Current evidence for central analgesic effects of NSAIDs: An overview of the literature. *Minerva Anestesiol,* 84(7): 865-870 (doi: 10.23736/S0375-9393.18.12607-1).

Wang J.Y., Chen R., Chen S.P., Gao Y.H., Zhang J.L., Feng X.M. et al. (2016) Electroacupuncture reduces the effects of acute noxious stimulation on the electrical activity of pain-related neurons in the

hippocampus of control and neuropathic pain rats. *Neural Plasticity,* 2016: 6521026 (doi: 10.1155/2016/6521026).
Ware M.A. (2011) Clearing the smoke around medical marijuana. *Clin Pharmacol Ther,* 90(6): 769-771 (doi: 10.1038/clpt.2011.241).
Welch S.P. (2009) Interaction of the cannabinoid and opioid systems in the modulation of nociception. *Intern Rev Psychiatry,* 21(2): 143–151 (doi: 10.1080/09540260902782794).
Welsch P, Petzke F, Klose P, Häuser W. (2019) Opioids for chronic osteoarthritis pain: An updated systematic review and meta-analysis of efficacy, tolerability and safety in randomized placebo-controlled studies of at least 4 weeks double-blind duration. *Eur J Pain,* 24(3): 497-517 (doi: 10.1002/ejp.1519).
Wiech K., Jbabdi S., Lin C. S., Andersson J., Tracey I. (2014) Differential structural and resting state connectivity between insular subdivisions and other pain-related brain regions. *Pain,* 155(10): 2047–2055 (doi: 10.1016/j.pain. 2014.07.009).
Wilson T.D., Valdivia S., Khan A., Ahn H.S., Adke A.P., Martinez Gonzalez S., Sugimura Y. K., Carrasquillo Y. (2019) Dual and opposing functions of the central amygdala in the modulation of pain. *Cell Rep,* 29(2): 332-346 (doi: 10.1016/j.celrep.2019.09.011).
Wilson-Poe A.R., Pocius E., Herschbach M., Morgan M.M. (2013) The periaqueductal gray contributes to bidirectional enhancement of antinociception between morphine and cannabinoids. *Pharmacol Biochem Behav,* 103(3): 444-449 (doi: 10.1016/j.pbb.2012.10.002).
Woodhams S.G., Chapman V., Finn D.P., Hohmann A.G., Neugebauer V. (2017) The cannabinoid system and pain. *Neuropharmacol,* 124: 105-120 (doi: 10.1016/j.neuropharm.2017.06.015).
Woolf C.J. (2020) Capturing novel non-opioid pain targets. *Biol Psychiatry,* 87(1): 74-81 (doi: 10.1016/j.biopsych.2019.06.017).
Wu Y., Yao X., Jiang Y., He X., Shao X., Du J., Shen Z., He Q., Fang J. (2017) Pain aversion and anxiety-like behavior occur at different times during the course of chronic inflammatory pain in rats. *J Pain Res,* 10: 2585–2593 (doi: 10.2147/JPR.S139679).
Xiao X., Zhang Y-Q. (2018) A new perspective on the anterior cingulate cortex and affective pain. *Neurosci Biobehav Rev,* 90: 200–211 (doi: 10.1016/j.neubiorev.2018.03.022)
Xu A., Larsen B., Baller E.B., Cobb Scott J., Sharma V., Adebimpe A., Basbaum A.I. et al. (2020) Convergent neural representations of experimentally-induced acute pain in healthy volunteers: A large-scale

fMRI meta-analysis. *Neurosci Biobehav Rev,* 112: 300-323 (doi: 10. 1016/j.neubiorev.2020.01.004).

Yam M.F., Loh Y.C., Tan C.S., Khadijah Adam S., Abdul Manan N., Basir R. (2018) General pathways of pain sensation and the major neurotransmitters involved in pain regulation. *Int J Mol Sci,* 19(8), pii: E2164 (doi: 10. 3390/ijms19082164).

Yang S., Chang M.C. (2019) Chronic pain: Structural and functional changes in brain structures and associated negative affective states. *Int J Mol Sci,* 20, 3130 (doi: 10.3390/ijms20133130).

Yarnitsky D. (2015). Role of endogenous pain modulation in chronic pain mechanisms and treatment. *Pain,* 156(4), Suppl. 1: S24–S31 (doi: 10. 1097/01.j.pain.0000460343.46847.58).

Zeilhofer H.U., Brune K. (2013) Cyclooxygenase inhibitors: Basic aspects. In: *Wall and Melzack's Textbook of Pain.* 6th ed., S.B. McMahon et al. (eds.), chap. 32. Philadelphia: Elsevier-Saunders, pp. 444-454.

Zhao X.Y., Liu M.G., Yuan D.L., Wang Y., He Y., Wang D.D. et al. (2009) Nociception-induced spatial and temporal plasticity of synaptic connection and function in the hippocampal formation of rats: a multi-electrode array recording. *Mol Pain,* 5: 55 (doi: 10.1186/1744-8069-5-55).

Zhuo M. (2016a) Neural mechanisms underlying anxiety–chronic pain interactions. *Trends Neurosci,* 39(3): 136-145 (doi: /10.1016/j.tins.2016. 01.006).

Zhuo M. (2016b) Contribution of synaptic plasticity in the insular cortex to chronic pain. *Neurosci,* 338(2): 220–229 (doi: 10.1016/j.neuroscience. 2016.08.014).

Zhuo M. (2019) Long-term cortical synaptic changes contribute to chronic pain and emotional disorders. *Neurosci Letters,* 702: 66-70 (doi: 10. 1016/j.neulet.2018.11.048).

Zimmermann M. (1983) Ethical guidelines for investigations of experimental pain in conscious animals. *Pain,* 16(2): 109–110 (doi: 10.1016/0304-3959(83)90201-4).

AUTHORS' CONTACT INFORMATION

Natia Tsagareli, PhD
Lab of Pain and Analgesia
Beritashvili Center of Experimental Biomedicine,
14 Gotua Street, 0160, Tbilisi, Georgia

Nana Tsiklauri, PhD
Lab of Pain and Analgesia
Beritashvili Center of Experimental Biomedicine,
14 Gotua Street, 0160, Tbilisi, Georgia

Merab G. Tsagareli, DSc, PhD
Head, Lab of Pain and Analgesia,
Ivane Beritashvili Center of Experimental Biomedicine
Beritashvili Center of Experimental Biomedicine,
14 Gotua Street, 0160, Tbilisi, Georgia
m.tsagareli@biomedicine.org.ge
m.tsagareli54@gmail.com

INDEX

A

affective-emotional aspects, vii
analgesia, vii, viii, 5, 18, 20, 25, 26, 28, 34, 39, 51, 56, 57, 61, 71, 74, 77, 80, 81, 82, 111, 124, 128, 129, 130, 132, 137, 139
anti-inflammatory, vii, x, 3, 29, 30, 39, 40, 41, 95, 124, 126, 131, 139
antinociceptive tolerance, v, vii, viii, 4, 43, 45, 58, 65, 66, 84, 86, 95, 113, 126, 129, 130, 135, 139
antipyretic, vii, 3, 41

B

brain limbic areas, v, viii, 4, 5, 98, 102, 111, 112, 113, 139

C

cannabinoid systems, v, viii, 4, 23, 24, 31, 34, 44, 83, 86, 112, 132
central amygdala, viii, 4, 85, 86, 113, 128, 138, 141
central nervous system (CNS), ix, 1, 3, 27, 31, 42, 96, 103, 108, 123, 127, 140
cingulate cortex, v, viii, ix, x, 2, 5, 6, 8, 9, 10, 14, 15, 45, 81, 102, 103, 104, 107, 112, 113, 126, 128, 132, 133, 134, 135, 139, 141

D

drug withdrawal syndrome, vii, 43, 44

F

formalin test, vii, x, 4, 34, 43, 51, 52, 58, 73, 84, 92, 101, 117, 131, 139

I

inflammation, vii, 3, 16, 39, 41, 42, 44, 61, 82, 97, 109, 110, 125, 132, 135, 136, 137
injury, iv, vii, ix, xi, 1, 10, 13, 14, 19, 20, 25, 31, 36, 95, 98, 99, 102, 105, 106, 137

insular cortex, v, viii, ix, x, xi, 4, 11, 12, 14, 16, 65, 83, 103, 112, 113, 123, 124, 128, 130, 131, 133, 135, 142

L

limbic system, vii, 2, 6, 8, 9, 13, 17, 19, 25, 45, 104, 105, 106, 111, 130

N

nervous system, ix, 1, 27, 127, 132, 140
nociceptive hyperalgesia, viii
nociceptors, vii, 1, 25, 95, 102
non-opioid antinociceptive tolerance, viii
non-opioid drugs, vii, 3, 43
non-steroidal anti-inflammatory drugs, vii, x, 2, 95, 124, 126, 139
NSAIDs, v, viii, x, 2, 3, 4, 40, 41, 42, 43, 44, 45, 46, 47, 48, 49, 50, 51, 52, 53, 54, 55, 56, 57, 58, 59, 60, 61, 62, 65, 66, 67, 68, 69, 70, 71, 72, 73, 74, 75, 76, 77, 78, 79, 80, 81, 82, 83, 85, 86, 87, 88, 89, 90, 91, 92, 93, 95, 96, 97, 112, 113,117, 118, 119, 126, 135, 138, 139, 140

O

opioid, v, vii, viii, ix, x, 2, 3, 4, 9, 17, 19, 21, 22, 23, 24, 25, 26, 27, 28, 29, 31, 34, 35, 36, 37, 39, 40, 41, 42, 43, 44, 48, 51, 52, 53, 54, 55, 57, 58, 63, 68, 70, 71, 73, 74, 76, 78, 82, 83, 84, 86, 87, 93, 95, 101, 109, 111, 112, 113, 116, 118, 119, 121, 122, 123, 124, 125, 127, 128, 129, 130, 131, 132, 133, 134, 135, 136, 137, 138, 139, 140, 141
opioid-like effect, vii, 42

P

pain receptors, vii, 1, 102
pain relief, vii, 23, 29, 37, 40, 99, 102, 111, 133
pain sensations, vii
physiological studies, vii, 130
public health, 1, 24

Q

quality of life, 1, 20

S

severe pain, 1, 23, 41